# Natural

## Healing

Marie D. Bajeux, RN, BS

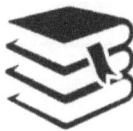

**BOOKS ACADEMY**
LEARNING LIFE FROM EVERY PAGE

**Books Academy LLC**

112 SW H K Dodgen Loop,

Temple, Texas 76504

Hotline: (254) 800-1189|


Ordering Information:

Quantity sales. Special discounts are available on quantity purchases by corporations, associations, and others. For details, contact the publisher at the address above.


Printed in the United States of America.


ISBN-13:     Softcover     978-1-964929-46-0

             eBook         978-1-964929-45-3

Library of Congress Control Number: 2024920102

# TABLE OF CONTENTS

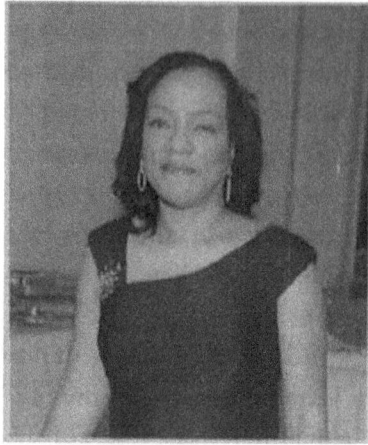

**G**ratitude is the perfect word to express my state of mind about my plant-based dietary lifestyle. I had an amazing experience while practicing this life-changing journey that started in 1999 and helped me regain my state of health. At 72, I feel blessed with the opportunity to see my 4 children becoming responsible adults. This is one of my greatest accomplishments in life. Over the past 20 years, my family has remained healthy through fitness exercises and daily consumption of organic fruits, vegetables, nuts, and seeds. Eventually, my children move out to start their journey of life and make their personal dietary choices. I make them realize that achieving good health is simply a choice between consuming nutritious live foods and unhealthy foods that are deficient in essential nutrients necessary to maintain wellness.

Many nutritionists advocate a plant-based lifestyle to not only heal but also detoxify the body and reduce inflammation which contributes to many chronic disorders such as diabetes, hypertension, and vascular disease. I wish others can experience that sense of wellness which can be achieved by nourishing the body with the vital nutrients that not only heal the body but also sustain good health.

My goal was to be able to help others improve and maintain their quality of life. In 2005, I received a BSN in Nursing which allowed me to teach my patients to incorporate high-fiber plant-based foods into their dietary regimen while complying with their meds. Adhering to healthy eating habits is not an easy task since most patients are reluctant to give up the foods they are accustomed to. My approach was to encourage and try to convince them that low-fat plant-based foods can delay, prevent, and perhaps eliminate the long-term complications associated with diabetes. I remember this 27-year-old obese male patient who suffered a heart attack and was diagnosed with heart disease, diabetes, and hypertension. He was very receptive, enthusiastic, and eager to start the health care plan designs to provide him with a new perspective of a better outlook on health. Six months later, he achieved his weight loss goal thereby lowering his a l c to a normal level. As a result, his healthcare provider was amazed with his progress and discontinued most of his meds. This life-changing experience can be achieved by anyone willing to make changes and adhere to healthy life choices that contribute to a state of good health.

I explored intermittent fasting which is useful for eliminating visceral fats which accumulate around the abdomen and other organs causing insulin resistance. Fortunately, a low-fat high-fiber plant dietary lifestyle combined with fitness exercise such as daily walking can be beneficial not only to achieve but also to maintain weight loss. Furthermore, unprocessed whole foods and low glycemic index foods of less than 55 such as apples, papaya, citrus fruits, vegetables, beans, etc. are excellent choices to control blood glucose.

Over the years, I was concerned about the side effects of premature aging. Research suggests that plants contain phytochemicals that can repair the body at the cellular level, delay the signs of aging, and sustain vitality. I am fortunate to have found and adhered to this healthy dietary lifestyle that helped me achieve my goal of aging gracefully. Everyone has the potential to experience similar results because the human body is very resilient whennourished with a variety of plant foods. I strongly believe that our Creator's plan for humans was to consume clean and healing foods since he placed our first parents in a beautiful exotic garden that provides a variety of plants designed to nourish the body and soul. Unfortunately, they stepped out of their boundaries by choosing the forbidden fruit which caused their downfall. People certainly suffer the consequences of their poor dietary choices which deprive the body of the necessary nutrients required to maintain good health and prevent disease.

I have to mention that children can benefit from eating healthy. They will get accustomed to proper nutrition and grow up to be healthy adults. The parent's role is to not only educate them on the importance of plant foods but also to provide them in their daily routine to promote wellness. I am convinced that the world will be a happier place if everyone starts practicing preventive medicine. Hippocrates, the father of medicine, taught humanity the most vital concept of natural healing by choosing plant foods as the best alternative means of medicine.

# INTRODUCTION

Numerous scientific evidences have shown that what we eat deeply compromises our start of health and longevity. Almost 70 percent of all diseases in the US are diet-related, according to the Surgeon General. The meat-centered Standard American Diet (SAD) has been linked to a staggering number of chronic conditions suffered by half of all adults in the US. More than 2,500 Americans die each day from heart disease, the leading killer of both women and men. Over 1.2 million Americans are diagnosed with cancer each year, and more than 500,000 die from this disease. Despite such horrifying findings many people continue to eat in ways that are extremely damaging to their health. They tend to accept the inevitable fact that soon or later they will succumb to some types of degenerative diseases.

We can no longer remain indifferent to those grim statistics if we expect to live a long and healthy life. It is absurd to wait until we get sick to start taking care of our bodies. The plain truth is we cannot depend on the healthcare system for disease prevention. It is not necessary to be a scientist to understand that our medical industry is not based on prevention. It is rather centered around pharmaceutical drugs and surgery for treatment once a disease has been identified. For the healthcare institution to remain lucrative, it cannot deal with illnesses from a preventive aspect. As a result, society failed to receive valuable health preventive information. Therefore, you must rely on your common sense and be willing to make a conscious dietary change to achieve wellness. Let's be realistic, it is not what your physician can do for you, it is rather what you can do for yourself to prevent those degenerative diseases from invading your body.

In 400 BC Hippocrates, the greatest philosopher during his time, said "Let food be your medicine and medicine be your food". After more than 2000 years, that ancient idea proved to be more powerful than ever. Eating the right food can indeed be a potent source of medicine. The healing properties of natural live foods have been proven to promote good health. Scientists worldwide have discovered various chemical compounds in fruits and vegetables that can alleviate and ward off disease. They have isolated various vitamins, minerals, enzymes, and phytochemical compounds, which are biologically active substances that play a significant role in disease prevention. These phytochemicals have been intensely tested and the result suggested that many of the diseases that plague our nation may caused by micronutrient deficiencies – that is lack of vitamins, minerals, enzymes, and phytochemical substances that are available only in plant foods. Unfortunately, these foods are lacking in the Standard American diet. According to the National Cancer Institute, less than 25 percent of Americans consume the proper foods that can reduce the risk of obesity, heart disease, cancer, and other chronic ailments. Many skeptics might think that despite all those diseases, the human average lifespan is 75 years. However, it is so depressing when you take a look around you to see and perhaps feel the anguish, agonizing pain, and despair so many people endured that make life is hopelessly miserable. The number of degenerative diseases is now reaching epidemic proportions. Too many people are aging prematurely and afflicted by health problems such as obesity, diabetes, cardiovascular diseases, headaches, weakness, arthritis, sinus, allergies, intestinal disorders, chronic fatigue, liver and kidney diseases – the list is endless. The sad truth is most of these excruciating pains are mainly related to poor dietary lifestyle and over-consumption of animal products and processed foods which are voided of the essential life-giving nutrients that support good health, and protect against diseases.

We can put an end to the epidemic of diet-related ailments and the despicable human suffering that is the legacy of the standard American diet. There are substantial medical pieces of evidence that people who eat a plant-based diet can dramatically reduce the risk of developing certain types of diseases. The China Health Project, which is the most extensive study of the correlation between diet and health, concluded that a low-fat plant diet can ultimately improve, prevent, and even eradicate many of the top diseases of our time. A diet rich in fruits, vegetables, nuts, and seeds contains a sufficient amount of vital nutrients such as antioxidants (beta carotene, vitamins C and E) phytochemicals, nourishing enzymes, and fiber that can help the body fight its own internal battle and ultimately heal itself.

You might be thinking that I sound as if I am trying to make a vegetarian out of everyone. The purpose of this book is not to persuade anyone to give up his or her current lifestyle to become a vegetarian. It is not my intention to tell you how to live your life or set up any type of dietary guidelines or restrictions. I am simply offering a wealth of suggestions based on my personal experiences so you can balance your lifestyle with pure, natural, nutritious living foods that will nurture and enrich not only your body but also your mind and spirit.

I am convinced that by choosing this book you are contemplating a positive dietary change that will not only help you. reclaim your health but also enhance your quality of life for years to come. Welcome to the delightful world of Healthy Living!

## TURNING POINT

**P**erhaps you are wondering why I became interested in nutrition. It is a long process that started in 1984 when I was going through the most critical health crisis of my life. In my early thirties, my health was failing. I started to suffer the consequences of the standard American diet. I was experiencing a lack of energy; I had a great deal of difficulty coping with my life. My symptoms were chronic fatigue, weakness, frequent urination, excessive thirst, insomnia, acne, sinus allergies, stomach pains, digestive disorders, mood swings, and depression. In the summer of 1984, my stomach pains became so severe that I had to check into an emergency room. The next morning, my appendicitis was removed. A few weeks later, I was diagnosed with the so-called Type 11 diabetes and was prescribed insulin to stabilize my blood glucose. Six months later, I went back to my doctor for a follow-up visit regarding my condition. He started to give me a lecture about my condition and the long-term complications associated with this condition. He told me that no matter what I do I can never regain my health since there is no cure for diabetes. That unscrupulous lecture left me in a state of shock. I could not believe how insensitive a doctor can be to a patient. He did not have any kind of compassion nor did he offer me even a ray of hope to alleviate my emotional turmoil. After I left his office, I was deeply devastated, angry, and saddened by the grim prospect that) will remain sick for the rest of my life. What frightened me the most was the idea that I would not be able to take care of my children. Faced with an uncertain future and the possibility of early death, I became withdrawn and emotionally unstable. I was really on the verge of a nervous breakdown. I spend most of my time in a deep depression. I kept wondering how I was ever going to feel well enough to get on with my life.

After a while, I got tired of feeling sorry for myself, for that state of sorrow instigated more grief than anything else. Thus, I decided that it was time to move on. Fear made me reassess a lifetime of mistakes under a new perspective. The fear of dying young intensified my strong will to live and encouraged me to look for an alternative course of action that could improve my health condition. I regained control of my emotions and decided to do some research regarding diabetes. I went to the bookstores, and luckily, I stumbled on a book titled "Reversing Diabetes" written by Julian M. Whitaker, M.D. This book renewed and strengthened my hope for better health. It contained the best educational materials about diabetes. The dietary guidelines were very easy for me to implement since I was already a vegetarian. I started a low calorie high complex carbohydrates diet combined with daily aerobic exercises, which helped me lose some excess weight, and stabilized my blood glucose. I monitored my blood glucose daily and consumed three small portion meals consisting of green vegetable salad, fruits, and grains.

During my illness, my doctor never asked me about my eating habits nor did he suggest any kind of physical activity that can improve my condition. However, he always seemed to be interested in what I do for a living and tried to make a connection between the stress of my job and health conditions. I have realized this is a skillful tactic to mislead a patient into believing that stress is the cause of most chronic disorders.

Well, I am proud to be among the millions of people around the world who have taken responsibility for their illnesses by educating themselves and changing their dietary lifestyles to reclaim their health.

I have realized that having a degenerative disease does not have to be a death sentence as my physician had tried to lead me to believe. I learned to treat my diabetes as a condition, not as a disease.

Most of the common ailments including the so-called diabetes are mainly related to poor dietary habits that can be improved and even reversed through proper diet and exercise. That concept is no longer a fantasy. Many conventional physicians have introduced in their practice Integrative medicine which regards certain diseases as potentially reversible through the remarkable power of the body to heal itself when nurtured with proper food, exercise, sunshine, rest, and massage.

My personal health experiences empowered me to explore a new horizon in my life. In my quest for more knowledge, I became fascinated with health and nutrition. Through reading so many health books, I have gained access to a wealth of beneficial educational information that has inspired me to write this book. I felt the willful need to share my experiences with others who may be going through the same trauma that had nearly destroyed my life. The idea of helping someone make a healthy dietary choice gave me the enthusiasm, energy, and passion to pursue my dream of becoming a writer. I committed to dedicate my time to educating others about a natural dietary lifestyle that will promote wellness rather than illness. I realized that the numerous health problems associated with obesity result from ignorance of how the human system works and the crucial role that proper nutrition plays in weight loss and disease prevention. Health is based upon the application of some natural laws. Failure to implement these principles will certainly cause damaging health repercussions. Therefore, it is in your best interest to gain nutritional wisdom to achieve physical, emotional, and spiritual health.

# DIABETES

According to the US Department of Health and Human Services, nearly 16 million people in the US suffer from diabetes which is the sixth leading cause of death in the nation.

A considerable amount of resources has been directed to its control and cure. And estimated $15 billion is spent yearly on this disease. However, all these researchers have not yet caused a significant impact on the increasing number of diabetic sufferers in this country. Although many researchers have established a correlation between diet and Type II diabetes, which afflicts 60 percent of diabetics, there are not enough resources and educational information available geared to prevent this chronic disorder. Since it is much easier to prevent any disease than to reverse it. In addition, the lack of dietary attention has resulted in the overwhelming unnecessary dangerous use of drug therapies such as hypoglycemic pills and insulin injections. In many cases, those drug treatments are often inappropriate and have the potential to cause more harm than good. Statistics indicate that most diabetic patients die from that condition. When the healthcare system recognizes the urgent need for the disease and starts advocating a healthy nutritional guideline designed to promote wellness, then we will eventually be able to prevent not only diabetes but also the host of degenerative disorders that plague our nation.

To prevent or manage diabetes, it is necessary to know what this condition is about, and the life-threatening risks associated with it. Diabetes is a chronic degenerative disorder that occurs when the pancreas loses its ability to produce insulin. This condition is commonly referred to as insulin-dependent juvenile diabetes (Type 1) because its symptoms appear during childhood or late in life if the pancreas is damaged or as a result of illness or injury. Insulin is a hormone that is essential for the proper absorption of glucose, which provides energy to the body's cells. When insulin is not available, excess glucose builds up in the bloodstream and not only becomes toxic but also spills over into the urine causing a sharp rise to the blood sugar level. This reaction causes the body to starve since the cells cannot get proper nourishment which must be provided by glucose to produce energy to carry out their normal functions. Symptoms of this condition include frequent urination, weight loss, chronic fatigue, weakness, and excessive thirst and hunger. Insulin injections are required to maintain normal blood sugar levels.

Since diet plays a major role in the prevention of diabetes, therefore, to avoid its potential health risks, it is imperative to eliminate from the diet all the unnatural foods that contribute poor health such as refined sugar products, processed foods, all animal products, dairy products, eggs, and processed oil. A low-calorie dietary regimen high in complex carbohydrates and fiber such as fresh fruits, vegetables, and sprouted seeds, combined with daily exercises can dramatically reduce the symptoms associated with this condition by regulating the release of glucose into the bloodstream. Fiber is essential to regulate glucose. It holds nutrients longer in the intestinal tract allowing a slower absorption rate, thereby, reducing blood fluctuation associated with poor diabetes control.

Many experts advocate that some nutritional supplements may also play an important role in diabetic therapy. There is evidence that vitamin C can help prevent blood vessel damage. B-complex vitamins help prevent nerve damage. Chromium may help metabolize blood sugar levels. Other therapeutic supplements include vitamin B-6, biotin, magnesium, vanadium, essential fatty acids, and flaxseed oil. In addition, spices such as cinnamon, clove, bay leaf, and turmeric may enhance insulin's ability to metabolize glucose.

While proper diet, exercise, nutritional supplements, and herbs may improve a diabetic's condition, diabetes is a very complex and serious condition that must be diagnosed with lab tests and managed with the help of a professional.

# THE CAUSE OF DIABETES

Everyone should be aware that there is nothing mysterious about the true nature and causes of diseases. The most common health symptoms revolve around the intestinal tract. The regular consumption of processed and cooked food lacks the live enzymes required for proper digestion. The pancreas, which is the most active gland in the digestive system, functions at its best when fresh raw foods are consumed. Natural foods do not leave toxic residues in the system. They are easier to digest since they contain live enzymes that facilitate the digestion, absorption, and elimination process. On the other hand, devitalized foods cause the pancreas not only to produce digestive enzymes but also to perform the task of converting them into their basic components. This extra activity depletes the system of its internal reserves of enzymes and wears down the pancreas. Furthermore, unnatural foods pass through the intestinal tract more slowly than live foods, thereby tend to ferment and putrefy causing the release of toxins into the body. The build-up of these poisonous wastes results in intestinal toxemia, which is the source of most illnesses including the so-called diabetes. A toxic body and a colon congested with morbid waste matter impair the cells of the pancreas's ability to produce insulin causing an intolerance of sugar in the body.

Many people who are afflicted by this condition found that the cleansing of the colon combined with a complete change of diet of fresh raw fruits and vegetables or whole juices can help manage their blood sugar level, thereby avoiding drug therapy. People who are obese and predisposed to develop symptoms of this condition need to change their eating patterns. The overconsumption of devitalized foods, which is a common problem associated with a high-fat cooked food diet, causes the pancreas to work overtime continuously. Years of overproduction of insulin may result in the complete shutdown of the pancreas, which becomes unable to produce the insulin required to turn foods into energy. Depending on the actual damage, the only way to get the production of insulin back to normal is by eating natural living foods that will assist the body in the detoxification process and the rejuvenation of the cells and tissues.

Most health symptoms have been shown to respond favorably to detoxification. It is vital to consume natural foods high in fiber to keep the walls of the colon clean and obtain live enzymes for effective digestion and assimilation of essential nutrients. Cooked foods more often go through the bloodstream as unsplit molecules that are stored as waste in many parts of the body. Living foods contain the enzymes required to split the molecules into simple substances so they can be readily utilized by the cells and tissues throughout the body.

# PERSONAL DIETARY CHANGES

D r. Whitaker's guidelines to reverse diabetes were valuable and very beneficial. They contributed enormously in helping me control my blood glucose and instigated a new positive outlook on health and nutrition as well. He focused primarily on the nutritional aspect of diabetes as the first mode of treatment to successfully manage this condition. I became very health-conscious and embraced a vegan dietary lifestyle. The basic four food groups in my household consisted of whole grains, legumes, fresh fruits, and vegetables. My family was strongly supportive and fascinated by this new healthy way of eating. It was like going on a culinary adventure. I bought some vegan cookbooks to ease the transition. Thus, my children were very anxious to experiment and explore the exotic world of delicious vegan cuisine. They also enjoyed chopping at the natural health food stores and the farmer's markets. However, as we started to incorporate daily fresh homemade fruit and vegetable juices into our diet regimen, we started consuming less cooked food. Our diet consisted of 80 percent raw foods.

I remained a vegan for about 7 years. However, in 1996, when I became aware of the detrimental effects of cooked food on health, my family and I engaged in a new experimental journey. In my quest for perfect health, I felt that it was time to take my dietary lifestyle to the highest level. I adopted a 100 percent food vegetarian diet, which has remarkably helped me achieve my optimum state of health. I must also attribute my wellness to my strong family support.

# THE ROLE OF PLANT ENZYMES

Through my incessant and intensive research about health and nutrition, I discovered that plant enzymes are essential in building and sustaining good health. These living microscopic elements can only be found in fresh raw foods and contribute to the breakdown of food in the digestive system. However, the process of cooking food at a temperature of at least 120 degrees even for a short period kills those living enzymes and destroys or alters most of the vitamins and minerals. Any item that is exposed to heat will undoubtedly start to break down and eventually turn to ashes. The same rational process applies to food. This concept can be easily verified by planting some live seeds and watering them, a few days later, they will be sprouted to life. When you try the same test with roasted seeds, they will simply rot. A dead seed cannot be sprouted because the enzymes are dead. The great harm of cooking is that it kills the life force in the food. For instance, notice how fresh and alive a raw broccoli looks compared to the wilted appearance of a cooked broccoli. Plant enzymes are chemical compounds that are very sensitive to heat and are deactivated through pasteurization, canning, or microwaving. The sun is the only source of energy that can cook food to a natural state of perfection.

Raw foods contain sufficient amounts of enzymes to ensure proper digestion. Foods that are devitalized through heat transformed into a foreign substance that is not only difficult to digest, but also puts a heavy load on the digestive system. You can perform your experiment by comparing a meal of fresh raw vegetables and a meal of the same kind of vegetables cooked. The raw meal leaves you feeling light, refreshed, and lively whereas the cooked meal generates a drowsy and sluggish feeling that lasts for hours. Instead of the efficient digestion that occurs with raw foods, the body is compelled to strive to digest the cooked foods, assimilate whatever nutrients it can, and dispose of the remaining toxic byproducts. The strenuous digestive process uses a great amount of energy from the body, which entails a decreased level of energy and a lethargic state.

It is important to understand the digestive process to value the vital role of plant enzymes. Humans digest food in different stages beginning in the mouth, moving to the stomach, and finally into the small intestines where all the nutrients are released into the bloodstream. At each stage, different enzymes break down different types of food. The body produces 22 digestive enzymes capable of digesting carbohydrates, sugars, proteins, and fats. However, raw foods contain different kinds of enzymes that can also digest foods. Plant enzymes function by predigesting the foods we eat in the stomach before they reach the stronger digestive juices. This digestive process preserves the body's internal enzyme supply for other functions necessary to maintain metabolic harmony. The body's use of its enzyme reserves for digestion depletes the immune system and impairs its ability to fight bacteria and viral infections. There is no wonder why so many people are suffering from chronic immune disorders. Eating live foods rich in natural enzymes ensures efficient digestion and preserves a considerable amount of energy. Therefore, the body can divert more energy into detoxifying, weight loss, and cell rejuvenation. Moreover, live foods such as fresh fruits, vegetables, nuts, and seeds infuse the body with a therapeutic dose of vitamins and minerals that contribute to the healing and strengthening of the body system.

Plant enzymes are not only essential for proper digestion of food but also increase the absorption of nutrients. They are necessary for every chemical reaction in the body. They are the elements that sustain life. Every vitamin, mineral, and hormone requires the help of enzymes to perform their particular function. Vitamins and mineral deficiency can be the result of a lack of enzyme production. Therefore, they play a significant role in promoting good health. I used to believe that we are what we eat, but based on the vital need for enzymes, I am strongly convinced that we are what we assimilate from the foods we consume. The body's ability to absorb and utilize the essential nutrients in food is the primary basis of optimum health. Daily inefficient digestion results in poor health, because the body is deprived of the life-giving nutrient supplies it requires to nurture the cells. Dead foods that are devitalized cannot possibly function the same way as live raw foods. Nevertheless, cooked foods that have lost their intrinsic nutritional value can maintain life in the human system. Unfortunately, they do so by gradually deteriorating the body's health and energy. Plant enzyme deficiency results from eating primarily denatured cooked foods. Years of cooked food intake that has been improperly digested generates an accumulation of toxic wastes in the colon producing a condition known as "toxemia" which can lead to numerous chronic health conditions.

Human beings are the only species on earth who have evolved into eating denatured cooked food. Animals who live on a natural diet don't suffer from any of the modern life health problems. The so-called degenerative disorders are relatively unknown in the wild where they live quite a long and healthy life. However, when they are domesticated, they develop similar ailments that afflict their owners simply because they are fed a diet that was not intended by nature.

The comforting news is that a proper diet of raw foods can bring tremendous health improvement to the diseases that we often think are genetic. Natural live foods enhance the body's vitality by providing the nutrients required to detoxify, strengthening, and healing the digestive system. Furthermore, as more nutrients become available to the system, the constant hungry feeling will subside which will cause a decrease in food intake. As those overburdened pounds begin to shed, most of your chronic symptoms will soon disappear. In time, the body will be revitalized and restored to new health, and you once again experience the wonderful feeling of wellness.

For years people have resorted to all kinds of quick fixes such as prescription drugs, and crash diets in a desperate attempt to regain their health or fight the battle of the bulge. If those methods fail to meet your expectations, then you may be willing to challenge a new approach that will undoubtedly help you in your quest for better health.

Before I adopted the raw food dietary lifestyle, I had heard so many incredible successful health testimonials from some raw foodists. I was anxious to investigate those claims. A few weeks after I started consuming a variety of raw foods, I began to notice a dramatic difference in how I look and feel. All my chronic conditions had gradually disappeared including my sinus allergy that I have been nursing for years, my acne cleared up to reveal a radiant complexion, my hair started to grow, and even my eyesight improved. As my digestive disorders vanished, I finally reached my ideal weight, as a result, I felt lighter, cleaner, and more energetic. As I started to experiment with foods that I never thought could be eaten raw such as beets or sweet potatoes, I kept wondering why anyone would want to cook these wonderful fruits and vegetables. Each one of them has a unique texture, crunch, juicy flavor, and freshness when eating in their natural state. I have suddenly realized that cooking and seasoning take away their natural flavor, and sweetness, and alter their natural chemical structure. The benefits of eating raw foods greatly surpass any other dietary lifestyle. The body becomes resilient when nurtured with live foods. Denatured cooked foods can only generate dead cells. A live food diet induces a live vibrant body full of energy and vitality.

I am supporting this dietary lifestyle simply because I have experienced its tremendous health benefits which have helped me achieve the optimum state of well-being. To some people, it might sound eccentric, extreme, or even idealistic. How ironic that living naturally has to be classified in such categories. Nevertheless, It takes inner strength, determination, and character to challenge and sustain such a revolutionary dietary lifestyle in a society that has been conditioned from birth to live on cooked foods. It is a daily ritual that everyone performs as an indispensable task. Some people may even feel uncomfortable just by thinking of giving up cooking. We become addicted to it our entire life evolves around cooked foods that people use as a source of comfort and entertainment. I realized that it would certainly be a formidable task to eradicate this eating pattern that has never been questioned and is generally accepted by everyone. However, there are substantial pieces of evidence that support the benefits of a diet consisting mainly of raw foods. As we look at other cultures these evidences are obvious. For instance, the Hunza people, who have been some of the most extensively studied vegetarians, are recognized for being the healthiest, longest-living people in the world. They have no diseases. Their high quality of life can only be attributed to their healthy diet consisting of mainly raw fruits and vegetables. It is a clear indication that live foods in their natural raw state must be the perfect diet for humankind.

Another good reason why I am advocating a raw food diet pertains to time and energy conservation. The most obvious reason why most people consume so many processed foods is to avoid going through the time-consuming chores of cooking and cleaning. Nevertheless, processed foods that require reheating in a microwave compound the ill effects of eating cooked foods not to mention the potential long-term hazards of this kind of radiation. The most nutritious raw meals can be easily prepared in a fraction of the time, thereby saving a great deal of time and energy. The simplicity of a raw food diet strongly appeals to me. When I am hungry, I no longer have to waste my time and energy in washing, chopping, and, cooking; with fruits, I just pluck, peel, and eat. There have been numerous debates regarding energy conservation in industry and households as well. The constant threat of air and water pollution and the potentially damaging effect of the ozone layer have prompted some advocates to search for new efficient ways to preserve energy. Considerable amounts of energy could be saved by not cooking, and the practice of consuming live foods would have tremendous benefits not only for the environment but also for our health. Consequently, our energy cost will decrease, while the energy supply from raw food intake will be maximized.

The greatest value of a raw food regimen besides being healthier is the inner change that results. Consequently, I became a stronger and more compassionate person with a more positive outlook on life. I have also acquired new aspirations, new interests, new visions, and new meaningful purpose in life. The habit of consuming pure, natural, clean foods brought me closer to nature, which revealed me to be more beautiful, appealing, and fascinating. I developed a great appreciation, respect, and love for nature that I never thought possible. I have also realized that living in harmony with nature provides a sense of relief and freedom from all forms of cooked food addiction and dead meat poisoning. This newfound liberation caused a deeper integration into the great life of nature and less of the baffled human world. It is such a delightful feeling that is impossible to believe unless you have experienced it. Some days, when I wake up in the morning, I feel so much joy and triumph over the conquest of all the common miseries of life such as headache, indigestion, excess weight, chronic fatigue, depression, and lethargy. At times this ecstasy causes a spontaneous vibration through my body generating a pleasant sensation. This experience convinces me that a pure living food dietary lifestyle is the most efficient way to achieve the connection of the body, mind, and spirit.

# THE VITAL NEED FOR FRUIT CONSUMPTION

**D**espite the consensus among nutritionists concerning the importance of fruit consumption, most people tend to eat fruit simply as an occasional treat. They fail to realize the positive health benefits that can be derived from consuming fruits regularly. Fruit is the most essential and nutritious food in the human diet. It contains a healthy combination of complex carbohydrates, fiber, fatty acids, natural sugars, enzymes, vitamins, and, minerals that the body requires to maintain good health. It is the ideal source of fiber, which plays a major role in helping control blood sugar levels, promoting regularity, and detoxifying the digestive system.

Fruit is the most natural and beautiful food on the planet. Almost everyone enjoys eating fruits, which come in an array of vibrant colors and graceful shapes that flatter the eyes. Each fruit has a distinctive aroma, a delightful flavor, and texture that is strongly appealing to humankind who seems to be instinctively attracted by them and enjoy eating in their raw natural state. It is a pleasant treat that has such a refreshing and cooling sensation on the body, especially during the hot weather season. Humans have an innate desire to indulge in fruits because that is what we are biologically and genetically designed to eat. Numerous studies of early primates' fossilized teeth suggest that they relied primarily on fruits for survival. They were not equipped with the proper tools required for hunting wild animals. Eventually, modern-day tools and the mastering of the skill to create fire have enabled mankind to sway from his original diet to become a carnivorous predator. We I should not continue to follow this destructive path, since we have experienced the ill effects of a meat-based diet. Nature supplies the best source of pure nutritious foods that have all the essential substances required by the body to sustain wellness.

The primary beneficial aspect of fruit consumption is the cleansing effect it produces on the body system due to its distilled water filled content, which has all the necessary nutrients capable of detoxifying but also revitalizing the human system.

All fruits contain about 80 percent cleansing-rich nutrient water. The body is constantly exposed to a variety of harmful elements such as pesticides, herbicides, food bacteria, fermented undigested protein residues, and chemical wastes. These pollutants invade our system, and as a result, they produce toxic wastes and acidity in the body. Therefore, it is crucial to dislodge and flush those accumulated wastes and neutralize the acidity, otherwise, the digestive tract will be clogged and unable to function efficiently. A toxic and acidic system may cause various health conditions such as excess weight, bloated, acne, cellulite, dark circles under the eyes premature aging, chronic fatigue, ulcers, nervousness, and constipation. Whole fresh fruits or juices are the mechanisms that can assist the body in cleansing and invigorating functions.

However, to reap the vital benefits of fresh fruits and juices, it is imperative to eat them on an empty stomach exclusively from awakening till noon, because the body needs to devote this time specifically to eliminate toxin residues without the burden of digesting food. When the digestive system is resting, energy is utilized in detoxification, rejuvenation, and weight loss. A light nutritious breakfast such as fruits yields a productive and energetic day, along with a feeling of lightness as opposed to the lethargic state that can result after indulging in a traditional breakfast of toast, bacon, and eggs or steak and potatoes. The body will certainly become fatigued resulting from the metabolic stress due to the substantial amount of energy those heavy meals require to be digested. It is rather ironic that a breakfast consumed for energy can deplete the body of energy. Believe it or not, any unhealthy and ill- combined meal does not provide energy, but use it instead.

Many years ago I learned about this natural hygiene concept in Harvey and Marilyn Diamond's book Fit for Life. I have incorporated this healthy habit into my dietary lifestyle, which has helped me not only maintain my weight but also provide the vitality I need to go through my daily routines.

Fruits, that are well chewed, are easier to digest and, thus do not require any energy. When eating on an empty stomach they take about 30 minutes to pass through the stomach into the intestines to release their vital nutrients. Dry fruits, dates, and bananas take about 45 minutes to clear up the stomach. Since fruits stay in the stomach for a short period, they should never be consumed mixed or following other foods. After feasting on a copious meal, it is customary to have a treat of fruit as dessert. A few minutes later you might experience some kind of discomfort or chest pain that may lead to heartburn or indigestion because the fruit is unable to go through the stomach into the intestines due to a previous meal. Consequently, your entire meal is putrefied and turns acid, you feel bloated and you end up burping that fruit for several hours. However, that discomfort could have been avoided by eating the fruit first and waiting 30 minutes before having the meal. That common practice of having a treat of fruit after a big meal violates the proper fruit consumption. Fruits can be eaten 3 hours after a properly combined meal, and about 8 hours after an ill-combined meal.

# HOW TO EAT FRUIT AND HOW MUCH

Fruit is the most important natural nourishment in our diet. They must be consumed in their raw fresh natural state to supply the body the essential nutrients that will contribute to its strength and general well-being. Any fruits that have been exposed to beat, altered, canned, or processed lose their active live nutrients specifically the vitamins, minerals, and enzymes which are very sensitive to beat. They become toxic acidic wastes that force the body to use a lot of energy to neutralize and excrete them out of the system. The same principle applies to fruit juices; they must be fresh and homemade. Processed and pasteurized fruit juices do not have any potent nutritional value because they are devitalized of the vital elements needed for cleansing and rejuvenating the system. They become concentrated acids that may cause potential damage from processed juices. It can benefit from fruits and juices intake only in their natural state of perfection.

When it comes to the amount of fruit one can eat, there is no limitation. Fresh fruits and juices can be consumed in generous amounts because they are not fattening. They are low in calories and will not add excess weight. On the contrary, fruit intake on an empty stomach from 8 AM till noon will promote weight loss. Their high fiber content will help control appetite by creating a feeling of fullness in the stomach that lasts for a long period. You must be aware that overeating may be the result of an unbalanced diet of very poor nutrients foods. When the body is not fed the proper foods, it can starve for specific nutrients, which may cause a constant hunger for more foods. Fruits are live foods that contain all the necessary substances that will satisfy the body's needs.

Human are frugivores who should take their nourishment from fruit trees. Fruits evolve from the tree root system combine with direct sunlight to produce a powerful complex nourishment. Mankind is perfectly suitable to eat fruits. Their digestion and absorption are easier than any other foods. The health benefits of fruits remarkably exceed many other foods since they do not leave toxic residues in the digestive tract. They are the cleansers and the revitalizers of the body. They are also the primary source of health and energy. Adding live foods to your dietary lifestyle will enhance your physical and mental performance; you will feel cleaner, lighter, and more energetic. Once you start experiencing the health benefits of fruit consumption, you will unravel nature's secret of weight loss, healing, health, energy, beauty, and happiness.

# THE POWER OF JUICING

During my avid quest for knowledge about health and nutrition. I came across The Encyclopedia of Healing Juices by John Heinerman. I was intrigued and fascinated by the remarkable therapeutic power of so many fruit and vegetable juices. I discovered the most effective and healthier way to nourish and replenish the body is by drinking fresh raw fruit and vegetable juices. For centuries, plant juices and extracts have been used for their healing properties. However, as we evolved into the modern-day era that practice became obsolete. Millions of people are becoming overly obsessed with consuming megadose of expensive vitamin supplements in the name of health and nutrition. They are unaware that a diet rich in live foods contains the most potent and natural source of supplements that provide all the essential nutrients in a balanced amount that the human body requires to maintain good health.

Juicing is the easiest and most efficient way to extract the essential nutrients stored within the cells of a plant. When fruits and vegetables are juiced, the fibrous cell walls burst open to release a pure concentrated live liquid that contains a rich supply of carbohydrates, fiber, natural sugars, amino acids, fatty acids, vitamins, minerals, and enzymes. These nutrients provide the body with the vital building blocks for cell rejuvenation. Since juices are predigested, their absorption requires a minimal amount of energy. Their life-giving nutrients are released instantly into the bloodstream to rejuvenate the cells and aid the body in its constant struggle of dissolving and eliminating toxic wastes.

**P**eople enjoy drinking some type of beverages. Rather than getting into the bad habit of drinking virulent liquids such as coffee, milk, processed juices, soda, beer, and alcohol, it is beneficial and healthier to consume fresh homemade fruit and vegetable juices. Their delicious flavors and high nutrient content make them the ideal beverage alternative to those toxic drinks. Fresh juices are pure and packed with live nutrients; they are free from additives and preservatives. Since they are homemade you know exactly what goes into them.

Another good reason for drinking fresh juices is to bypass the digestive process. Solid foods require several hours to digest before their nutrients become available to the cells and tissues of the body. When we eat whole fruits and vegetables, the body must extract the liquid from the fiber. However, when we consume juices, the digestive process is eliminated. The vital nutrients are absorbed into the bloodstream in a matter of minutes. Almost everyone entertains the idea of drinking natural juices and can certainly benefit from them. By nourishing the body with the essential elements of life including vitamins, minerals, and live enzymes, you are ensuring the state of health of every cell and organ in your system. Incorporating live juices into your diet will eliminate the need to take vitamin supplements, which are toxic substances that undermine your state of health. Fresh juices supply the body with a natural healthful balanced nutrition that cannot be duplicated in any way by scientific technology. Vitamin supplements are substances that are mass-produced and designed to profit at the expense of human health. Once you start drinking fresh juices you will undoubtedly experience the wonders of their healing powers.

Juices can be beneficial for those people who lost their ability to chew well enough to break down the cell walls of certain fruits and vegetables. They tend to break down and assimilate more slowly in the system. In addition, vegetables in general are difficult to digest and absorb by the digestive system when eaten whole. Therefore, consuming their juices eases the digestion and assimilation process, and ensures that the full benefits of their nutrients are readily available.

Vegetable juices are essential in a healthy dietary regimen. They are rich in complex Carbohydrates, vitamins, and minerals necessary to maintain strong healthy muscles, bones, and tissues. It is important to drink at least two glasses of vegetable juices daily. Orange and yellow vegetables are a good source of beta-carotene, a substance that the body converts into vitamin A. Green leafy vegetables not only contain beta-carotene and vitamin C, but also are rich in magnesium, potassium, calcium, iron, and chlorophyll, which is another element that may protect against cancer.

Vegetable and fruit juices should never be mixed. The only exceptions are apples and carrots. "Most vegetables are alkaline and high in mineral salts, and most fruits are acidic and contain a lot of natural sugars. The body processes alkaline food one way and handles acid another way. Also, minerals undergo a special chelation process within the body so they can be properly stored where needed the most. On the other hand, carbohydrates are converted to fuel and "burned" within the system to produce energy and strength. When mineral-rich vegetables and sweet fruit juices are mixed, they often produce intestinal discomfort and chemical disturbance within the body. Green juices derived from vegetables such as lettuce, kale, spinach, broccoli, or cabbage are very concentrated and potent for the body to handle. They should not be consumed pure, they must be diluted with either carrot or apple juice to decrease their strength and make them more appetizing.

# HEALTH BENEFITS OF JUICES

Fresh fruit and vegetable juices play a powerful role in sustaining good health. They provide a nutritional foundation that assists the human system in the cell regeneration process, thereby promoting healthy muscles, tissues, glands, and organs. The abundance of live enzymes and other nutrients in raw fresh foods flush out the deadly body toxins, leaving you feeling cleaned, refreshed, and revitalized. Juices can also help prevent and alleviate certain chronic ailments, stimulate the immune system, lower blood pressure, and protect the body from potentially harmful atmospheric substances. Furthermore, live foods will make your skin radiant, your hair shine, your breath fresh, and regulate your entire system.

Research has shown that certain substances found in fruits and vegetables can inhibit the harmful effects of carcinogen agents in the body. For instance, vitamin such as beta-carotene plays a prominent role in the prevention of many types of cancer including breast, colon, and rectal cancer. Studies have shown that it can also lower the risk of coronary disease, and high blood pressure. Beta-carotene functions as an antioxidant that can neutralize harmful molecules known as free radicals. Therefore, it is vital to consume more fruit and vegetable juices for maximum protection against degenerative diseases. Good sources of beta-carotene include carrots, broccoli, cabbage, cauliflower, spinach, green, kale, Brussels sprouts, and watercress. Whole juices are the ideal source of fiber, which is an essential component of human health. An adequate amount of fiber in the diet can help protect against cancer and heart diseases. Fiber may also improve bowel function, cleanse the colon, reduce blood pressure, and lower cholesterol. Therefore, it is crucial to consume the juices with the fiber. In addition, drinking pure juice without fiber can create a blood sugar imbalance in the system. Pure juices that are high in natural sugar content will cause a sharp rise in the blood sugar level especially if a person is afflicted with diabetes or hypoglycemia which are the most common blood glucose condition. The fiber of fruits and vegetables is the most perfect mechanism that allows their sugar and nutrients to be slowly absorbed into the bloodstream, thereby regulating and stabilizing the blood glucose level.

To prevent a sudden sugar surge from occurring in the body, and the loss of dietary fiber which is an important part of juicing, you will need to consider investing in a "blender juicer," which can puree or liquefy the pulp, skin, and seeds. Unlike other juicers, which separate the juice from the pulp, the blender juicer makes smooth nutritious drinks loaded with fiber. When it comes to puree juicing, among all the juicers in the market, The Vita-Mix Total Nutrition Center unit was tested the best by the Prevention Health Magazines Food Center. It is very efficient and versatile, it does not require any assembly, and can easily be cleaned by simply rinsing out the container with soap and hot water. It is a very powerful machine that produces delicious fruit smoothies and luscious juices in a fraction of the time required by other machines, thereby saving considerable time not only in the actual juicing but also in the final cleanup.

For people who never experienced the joy of juicing, it will be a pleasant and exotic adventure. Using a blender juicer will make juicing an easy and simple task. It is preferable to use certified organically grown products that are free of pesticides. But, if you are unable to find organic harvest, you may use regular produce, however, it is important to scrub and wash them thoroughly with a biodegradable cleanser designed to remove the pesticides, herbicides, and other chemical residues on their surface. These cleansers are sold at health food stores. It is a good habit to clean the produce as soon as you come home from the supermarket, dry and store it in a plastic bag, so it is ready to be juiced. If you prefer, you may add some herbs such as cinnamon, nutmeg, ginger, and vanilla to enhance the juice's flavor.

The best way to start your day is to drink a glass of fresh juice in the morning. It has a refreshing and stimulating effect on the body. One of my favorite morning juices consists of a combination of apple, parsley, carrot, and celery, which is very energizing and beneficial for relieving sinus allergy symptoms. Another of my preferred drinks is apple, carrot, and banana with a sprinkle of cinnamon, some days I would add a small parsnip, which is not only an excellent appetite suppressant, but also helps improve the skin, hair, and nail condition. You should drink at least four glasses of juice a day. To reap the full benefits of juices they must be consumed immediately after juicing to avoid losing their potent nutrients. Remember to drink slowly mixing the juices with your saliva. Gulping or drinking too fast may cause a sudden rise in the blood glucose level. It is very convenient to sip the juices with a straw for a slower intake.

Be aware that it is never too late to start eating healthy and living well. I consider myself very fortunate to be able to achieve and maintain an excellent state of health that I never thought possible. Although I am in my late forties, I feel and look better than when I was in my thirties. I am convinced that the dietary habit of eating and drinking fresh, live, natural foods combined with daily exercises contribute to my healthy, vibrant, and energetic body. I have concluded that the ideal and effective way to achieve good health is to incorporate more live foods into the diet. After a few weeks of consuming fresh juices, you will experience an immense surge of energy. Your system will be detoxified and you will feel the need to eat only fresh live foods. As a result, you will probably lose the craving for unnatural foods. You will go to the produce aisle of the supermarket with a new interest in mind, visualizing new juice recipes. You will feel a strong desire to explore the world of living foods because you will be attracted to them. That is what being on a natural and healthy dietary regimen is all about. You will develop a nutritional concern combined with a sense of health consciousness that arises as you come to realize the benefits and the inner pleasure of feeling and looking great.

Most people always have the intense desire to look their best. Physical attractiveness seems to be their number one priority. Although the passing of time may fade away our youthfulness, we never quite lose the longing to look our best. Those expensive vitamin pills, facial treatments, beauty lotions, and rejuvenation creams always fail to meet our expectations. Women go through so many torments to improve their skin appearance, however, looking younger is easily within our reach. Live foods will undoubtedly nurture and replenish your skin from the inside out. Fresh fruit and vegetable juices are rich with all the required nutrients that can reverse and delay the signs of aging. The key to radiant skin is no longer a mystery. All the products you need to maintain or improve your skin condition are in the produce aisle of your supermarket. You simply have to get accustomed to them until you develop a passion for them.

I strongly encourage you to start juicing right away. It will be such a rewarding experience. It is the most effective way to maintain or lose weight without depriving your body of the necessary nutrients required to sustain wellness. The high fiber content in puree juices helps control your weight by providing added bulk that fills your stomach and curbs your appetite. Fresh fruits and vegetables are fat-free, low in calories, and can be added as a supplement to your regular meals. They are the only beverages that are beneficial to your health and supply vital energy, improve your stamina, and enliven your spirit as well.

The key to good health resides in the live nourishing enzymes, the life energy, and the various vitamins and minerals content of raw foods that can produce live cells. Health starts at the cellular level; thus, living cells must be nourished by living foods. Cooked fruits and vegetables or any cooked foods for that matter are dead foods that have lost their natural goodness and innate nutritional benefits. Therefore, they can only disintegrate the cellular system, and undermine the body's health. Live food consumption is a delightful path to natural living. Incorporating live fresh uices into your dietary lifestyle is a giant step toward "Healthy Living."

# THE CONCEPT OF DETOXIFICATION

Your body is the sanctuary in which you live. Therefore, it requires meticulous attention to remain in prime condition. Every physical, mental, and spiritual function depends on the particular care you give to your body. The type and quality of food you ingest in your system is extremely vital to every aspect of your well-being. Your body is at the mercy of various toxic chemicals and pollutants in the atmosphere, food, water, and soil. People carry in their system a virulent cocktail derived from industrial chemicals, herbicides, pesticides, food additives, heavy metals, alcohol, tobacco, and the residues of pharmaceutical and narcotic drugs. These toxic substances are building in the human system faster than they are eliminated, thereby causing extensive health damage. Proper nutrition not only rejuvenates and rebuilds the cells and tissues which are the components of the physical body but also assists in the natural process of eliminating the toxic wastes, the dead cell proteins, and the undigested food residues from the system to prevent their fermentation and putrefaction.

The proper elimination of undigested food and other waste products is as vital as efficient digestion and assimilation. When those wastes accumulate and remain in the system, they ferment, putrefy, permeate the colon walls, and produce a toxic and acidic condition. Many people fail to realize the importance of efficient elimination. Everyone has a certain level of tolerance that may not be exceeded to remain healthy. If the amount of toxins remains below that level, then the body can usually adapt and get rid of them. However, when the system is overloaded, the body's defense system malfunctions causing various health symptoms that indicate the body's need to be detoxified. Sickness is simply nature's warning sign that the body is filled with toxic wastes and needs to be detoxified.

Detoxification is the body's natural process of eliminating and neutralizing deadly toxins via the bowel, bladder, lungs, and skin. However, it is crucial to consume the proper food for this process to occur efficiently and continuously as well. Fresh raw fruits and vegetables will supply the body with the required nutrients to adequately perform the elimination process by removing toxic matters, reinvigorating the digestive system, and preventing chronic diseases. The modern-day diet with excess animal protein and fats, devitalized starches, and processed and cooked foods inhibits the body's natural functions of self-cleansing and self-healing abilities. Since we consume so many foods that have been altered from their natural state and are difficult to digest and assimilate the undigested food remains as residues in the colon and become toxic. Rather than providing nourishment to the various nerves, muscles, cells, and tissues of the colon walls, denatured foods can inevitably cause starvation of the system. The accumulation of toxic wastes in the system generates a condition known as toxemia. This condition occurs primarily through normal body function and also by the leftover food particles that are not properly used. In addition, toxins produce an acid buildup in the body which strives to neutralize this condition by retaining excess water causing bloating and excess weight. A toxic and acidic colon that results from the accumulation of wastes that are corrupted in the colon seriously compromises the absorption of vital nutrients required by the body to protect and fight off diseases. Consequently, when a colon contains toxic substances, any nutritional elements would pass through the bloodstream as polluted products. If untreated toxemia may lead to numerous chronic degenerative conditions including obesity, chronic fatigue, stress, insomnia, headache, digestive disorders, constipation, immune disorders, acne, mood swings, arthritis, cancer, and cardiovascular diseases, to name just a few.

You certainly have experienced the repulsive odor that emerges from the decomposed carcass of a dead animal and the worm infestation that it produces. The same process occurs in humans when dead protein cells and toxic products remain in the colon for longer than necessary, thus causing the same offensive odor to emanate from the bowels which meat eaters are so familiar with. Nature requires that the human digestive be cleansed regularly to avoid any health disintegration. Failure to comply with natural laws is like allowing a collection of garbage to gather in your home, causing putrid, obnoxious, and unhealthy gas to be released into the air.

A congested colon means that constipation is present in the system. That chronic condition is the primary source of nearly every ailment afflicted mankind. Constipation has a tremendous impact on the health of the colon upon which the wellness of the body depends almost entirely. The colon is interrelated to every cell and tissue in the body and supplies their vital nourishment.

The human body must be nurtured to live. The cells and tissues that constitute the physical anatomy are live organisms with a remarkable degree of resilience. To be replenished and regenerated, they must be nourished by live-giving elements that can only be found in fresh raw natural foods. These foods also contain special substances whose ultimate task is to ensure efficient cleansing and quick removal of dead cell proteins and waste products before they become toxic. The digestive system requires bulk in the form of fiber or roughage for efficient digestion. Those fibers are the ideal transport system since they are naturally highly magnetized and have a sweeping effect on the intestine. However, excess cooked food strains the digestive system and simply passes through the colon where it becomes toxic waste. These denatured foods fail to provide any nutritional benefits to the body leaving a coating that smears the inner walls of the colon. As the coating gradually thickens to a narrow opening packed with toxins, you unconsciously starve your body, and the result manifests in obesity and illnesses, which are the direct result of indulging in denatured cooked foods that allow the colon to remain cluttered with corruption.

The colon is the human sewage system; therefore, it is a natural breeding ground for bacteria. It carries two types of bacteria: the healthy- friendly bacteria known as bacilli coli, and the pathogenic or disease- producing type. In a clean healthy environment, the friendly bacteria will fight the harmful ones. However, when the colon is toxic, the pathogenic bacteria intensify resulting in numerous health conditions. This condition contributes to the infiltration of poisonous products into the bloodstream. For instance, skin disorders such as pimples or acne are an indication that poisonous bacteria have infected the blood supply. It is crucial to nourish the body the living foods that will not clog the digestive tract and help maintain a healthy intestinal flora.

You should be aware that the toxins in your body may have taken several years to accumulate, therefore, you cannot expect the detoxification process to occur hastily. Depending on the toxicity of the system, it might take several months or even years to completely remove all the impurities from the body. When you start consuming fresh fruit in the morning on an empty stomach, you may experience some kinds of discomfort the first few days. As your body is trying to adjust to this new dietary style, symptoms such as headache, bloating, flatulence, and weakness may occur, along with the passing of loose stools as the water-filled nutrient content of fruits start stirring up, washing, and flushing out the impacted fecal matters from the colon walls. After a few days, you will start feeling lighter, refreshed, and more energetic.

## BENEFIT OF DETOXICATION

A toxic or acidic system inhibits the optimum functions of the cells and tissues. The cleansing of toxins and waste matter will restore their functions and vitality. A detoxification process through fresh fruits and vegetables or whole juices will reinvigorate the body and restore health. You will experience greater mental clarity, an increased energy level, and a reduction of stress on the immune system. Other benefits include lower blood pressure and cholesterol levels. Detoxification helps maintain the proper function of the intestinal flora and will enhance its natural ability to resist infections, allergies, as well as skin 9 disorders. A clean system is the key to achieving successful and permanent weight loss since the body can supply the energy necessary to eliminate excess weight.

The health of the body primarily depends on the condition of the colon. Most diseases originate in the colon, which is directly related to every cell and tissue in the body. Toxicity is the primary source of most diseases. Every function in our system requires energy. A clean colon releases more energy that the body can utilize for other important functions such as repairing and maintaining cells and tissues and weight loss. A clean system also enhances the absorption of live nutrients necessary to promote good health and prevent chronic diseases.

It is imperative to live in harmony with nature by adopting a simple and natural lifetime approach perfectly suitable to efficiently assist the body in carrying out its vital functions. This is what the concept of natural hygiene is about. Its basic foundation is that mankind has a marvelous healing power that can be perpetuated by complying with the laws of nature. Its primary goal is to nurture and replenish the system with pure natural living elements that can help the body in its ingenious capability of self-cleaning, self-healing, and self-maintaining functions.

Detoxification is a lifetime habit that can easily be incorporated into your dietary lifestyle. A daily consumption of 80% of live foods will keep the colon in good condition and provide the rich nutrients to sustain good health. It is a daily routine that must be developed to ensure wellness and longevity as well. It does not require any special foods, no calorie counting, and no food restriction. It is the most ideal and efficient tool to maintain and lose weight.

There are several detoxification procedures available including distilled water fasting, specific diets, chelation therapy, colon irrigation, and hyperthermia. However, juice or water fasting, and daily fruit and vegetable consumption are the safest, easiest, and most natural methods to detoxify the body. Distilled water fasting is the greatest cleanser, purifier, and healer of the body. Three to ten days of water fasting will expel the toxic wastes and poisonous substances buildup in the body. Fasting gives the system a physiological rest that allows the body to use its vital force to eliminate the deadly toxins to help it become clean, pure, and healthy. It generates a storehouse of energy; consequently, you will feel vigorous, lively, vibrant, and healthy. A powerful detoxifying cocktail that combines equal parts of spinach, parsley, and apple juice will cleanse and rejuvenate the intestinal system. Drink three cups a day on an empty stomach every four hours. A glass of warm water mixed with one fresh lemon juice upon arising is an excellent morning drink that will flush your kidneys and liver.

Many studies confirm the vital significance of vitamin C in healing and maintaining health. There is also a correlation between vitamin C and toxicity in the body. A deficiency in vitamin C not only increases the body's potential harm from environmental pollutants but also inhibits the body's natural detoxification process. Vitamin C is a very potent detoxification agent that can neutralize and destroy certain toxins in the system.

In addition, it helps maintain the connective tissue system of the body which is the bond that holds the cells, the various organs, and glands in their proper place. Since the body cannot produce vitamin C, it must be obtained daily from the food we eat. The richest sources of vitamin C include rosehip, grapefruit, lemon, lime, orange, tangerine, cherries, and kiwi. Although most fresh fruits and vegetables have varying amounts of ascorbic acid.

A daily consumption of fresh fruit and vegetable juices will detoxify the colon to prevent the degenerative condition associated with toxemia and improve your chances of living a long and healthy life. Detoxification is the most effective mechanism to prevent or even eradicate the potential risk of certain life-threatening diseases. It is also a way to alleviate and heal many early health conditions. There is an urgent need to educate people about the danger associated with toxemia, and the vital need to make the necessary dietary changes that can help improve or prevent their health problems. Many alternative healthcare experts have been using various detoxification therapies to treat their patients. However, more emphasis should be on preventive measures rather than on disease control. There is an absolute necessity to address this issue before the deterioration of the internal vital organs, and health disturbances.

Your body deserves the best possible care to function at its highest level of performance, unconstrained by toxins and excess weight. There is a slim and energetic body buried beneath those layers of fat longing to emerge. The body you have been incessantly fantasizing about, with the original contour that nature intended and designed for you to have. Why not make a conscious dietary decision to allow that beautiful silhouette to become the new you? You are the only one who can make it happen by living under the laws of nature. You have the principles and the means to achieve that goal. You must gain the wisdom to put them into practice to reach your ideal weight dream that is long overdue. Your body is yearning for nutrient-rich living foods that have the therapeutic power to cleanse, condition, and revitalize the system to help it regain the strength and energy necessary for a successful weight loss achievement. A clean colon will contribute to better health and an increase in vitality, which are the prerequisites to a vibrant life.

# THE BODY'S ESSENTIAL NUTRIENTS

As we cross the bridge to the new Millennium, it is time to reevaluate our dietary lifestyle and perhaps focus on a natural way to nourish the body to achieve a general feeling of well-being. For years, we have learned a great deal about animal products that carry parasites and bacteria and are loaded with sulfa drugs, antibiotics, growth hormones, and steroids. We also have witnessed and even experienced the tremendous health threats associated with the consumption of animal proteins and dairy products. However, we are reluctant to give up these foods which have such a damaging effect on the human body. The need to satisfy our cravings outweighs their health consequences. Nevertheless, there is no doubt that our state of health strongly reflects our genetic reaction to the way we eat and care for our bodies. In other words, the way we feel is directly related to our food consumption. Of course, when we are young and healthy, we may not realize or even feel the ill effects of an animal-based diet and cooked food consumption. However, years of ingesting unnatural and devitalized foods will inevitably intoxify the body. You will most likely be subjected to some potential chronic health conditions that will impoverish your quality of life. You will eventually have to make frequent visits to your doctor and the drug store for your constant need for prescription refills, not to mention the lingering pain that can inflict so much agony on the body and soul as well.

The contemplation of such a grim future can be very disturbing. I am certain that everyone would love to enjoy a vigorous life even in old age. Most people envision the idea of living a long, productive, and healthy life free from pain, free from popping up prescription pills that very often prolong suffering or cause premature death. Keep in mind that regaining your state of health can be a formidable task since some health conditions can be irreversible. Therefore, it is imperative to take some simple course of preventive actions. Since improper diet is the primary cause of most health afflictions, accordingly, a dietary lifestyle change is the most effective treatment to relieve or prevent most degenerative chronic ailments. Rather than continuously focusing on controlling the effects of a condition, the elimination of the cause of a disease will consequently allow the body to heal itself. Although the human body is a very complex machine, it can be simple and easy to manage if one is willing to live by the laws of nature. Vitality, health, and energy which are the essence of life can be within the reach of everyone. The body is constantly striving to fight off the negative external forces to remain healthy, nevertheless, the way we live impedes this process. Living organisms must be nurtured and preserved with living elements. Live cells and tissues require essential nutrients found in live foods for detoxification, rejuvenation, maintenance, repair, reproduction, and disease prevention. The efficiency of these physiological functions depends entirely on your dietary choices. Some basic nutritional principles will clarify this concept.

The prerequisite to wellness is to primarily satisfy the body's nutritional requirements. When you become conscious of your body's need for essential nutrients, making a healthful dietary choice will be an easy task. Nutrients are substances that are essential for life. They are required for every bodily function including the maintenance of healthy cells and body tissues. A balanced nutrition is necessary to provide your body with these vital nutrients. It is fairly simple to put into practice, as long as you keep in mind that mankind has no nutritional needs for the flesh and milk of any animals. Nature has provided a wealth of plant foods that can supply everyone with all the essential health-giving nutrients: carbohydrates, oil, water, vitamins, minerals, and proteins. When you supply your body an adequate amount of these nutrients from natural live foods you will be on your way to a clean state of health.

# CARBOHYDRATES

A high-performance racing car will require premium fuel to run efficiently. The human body has the same needs, and its ideal source of fuel is carbohydrates. They are the most potent source of energy that the body requires to perform adequately. Carbohydrates contain dietary nutrients including sugars, starches, and fiber, and are the body's main source of energy. They are sugar compounds from plants that are made of carbon and water which the digestive system process into fuel.

Carbohydrates break down fats and team up with protein to generate compounds that are vital for fighting infections, producing hormones, renewing cells, repairing wounds, and maintaining healthy skin, bones, nails, and hair. They are classified as simple or complex depending on their chemical structure. Both kinds contain four calories per gram and are digested into a blood sugar known as glucose, which the body uses as fuel for work or exercise.

Simple carbohydrates are refined sugars such as granulated white table sugar, fruit juices, maple syrup, and molasses, which contain very few essential vitamins and minerals. Refined sugar is widely used in soft drinks, candy, and other processed foods; they are high in fat and depleted of nutrients. Simple sugar supplies glucose to the body and absorbs quickly in the bloodstream to provide energy. However, excessive amounts of refined sugar in the diet can cause tooth decay, promote obesity, and raise blood sugar levels.

The best forms of simple carbohydrates are natural sugars known as fructose, which is found in fruits and contains essential nutrients.

Complex carbohydrates commonly referred to as starches also supply the body with glucose. They are found in whole grains, beans, fruits, and vegetables. Complex carbohydrates are simply chains of single sugar molecules that bond together to make long branching chains. Physical processes transform these simple sugars into energy to provide fuel for the body's functions. They take longer to digest since the digestive system must break them into simple sugars. This process slows down the absorption of the glucose into the bloodstream.

I used to believe that starches were the perfect food for humans. For years, nutritionists have been advocating the consumption of starches as the ideal source of energy. As a result, they play a dominant role in the human diet. However, when I became a raw foodist, I discovered that grains that require cooking before consumption are not fit for human consumption, and do not satisfy the body's requirements for essential nutrients. Grains are tasteless foods that cannot be consumed in their natural raw state. They require cooking which kills the living enzymes and vitamins necessary for proper digestion. The body must use its source of reserve nutrients to convert them into energy. This process not only cause nutrient deficiency but also impedes various body functions.

Starches contain excessive acid-forming minerals. The relative acidity or alkalinity of foods is critical to diet and health. The human system has a pH balance, which reflects the level of acidity or alkalinity. Infusing the body with a toxic dose of acid can cause serious health threats. Acidic foods can interfere with the proper functioning of the digestive system. The pH of the blood always remains n the alkaline side. To maintain an alkaline blood pH level, it is vital to eliminate starches from the diet.

Chemists have isolated fifteen separate opioids in wheat that can cause the same body reaction as opium, which is a well-known addictive and sedative compound. Since energy is the essence of life, any foods that have addictive properties, and slow down mental and physical abilities should be omitted from the diet.

The consumption of starch has been associated with various health conditions. But the most common ill effect is congestion. The gluten in most starchy foods promotes excess mucus. The body reacts to starch consumption by producing mucus as a way of protection and expelling the gluten out of the system. In addition, the starch molecule is not soluble in water. Thus, it passes through the system as a solid molecule that the body cannot utilize and tries to eliminate as toxins. The accumulation of these molecules smears the walls of the intestines like a paste that the body expels as purulent substances through the skin. Thereby, causing various skin inflammations such as acne, pimples, or rashes.

Starches are unnatural foods that do not provide the nutrients necessary to promote good health and require more energy to digest. If a human was physiologically designed to consume grains, we would be adapted to ingest them in their raw natural state. Cooking starches to make them palatable and digestible stripped them of their nutritional value, leaving only the empty calories. When we take a close look at nature, we will find that only a few species of birds and insects eat grains. Primates such as gorillas, and chimpanzees, which have incredible strength and closely resemble humans, do not consume grains. There are primarily frugivores.

Americans consume excessive amounts of starches. The most alarming concern is that most of these starches are refined grains loaded with sugar and fat which are empty-calorie foods that promote obesity and intoxify the body. Those denatured foods are difficult to digest; they weaken the immune system and debilitate the body. The best choices of nutritious carbohydrates include fruits, vegetables, sprouted seeds, and raw nuts. They must be consumed in their raw natural state. They are packed with enzymes, vitamins, minerals, amino acids, fiber, and fatty acids, and provide proficient energy to the body to sustain a rigorous lifestyle.

# FIBER

C arbohydrates not only supply efficient energy to the body but also provide fibers, the indigestible substance exclusively found in plant foods that are essential for the proper function of the human intestines. They are prerequisites for a healthy elimination process. Fibers can be best described as the transport system of the digestive tract that carries waste products out of the colon. They help relieve constipation, lower cholesterol, regulate blood glucose, prevent colon cancer, aid in weight loss, and ensure the proper functioning of the digestive system. Fivers are found in fruits, vegetables, nuts, and seeds. They are classified as soluble and insoluble. Many plants contain both types of fibers.

Soluble fibers form a gel in the colon, which slows down the movement of foods through the intestines. This process delays the absorption of nutrients. They cause glucose to absorb gradually into the bloodstream to regulate the blood sugar level of diabetics. They also lower cholesterol by washing out bile acids in the digestive tract to prevent them from being converted into cholesterol. Soluble fibers are found in plants high in pectin and gum such as apples, citrus fruits, flaxseeds, and psyllium.

Insoluble fibers have tremendous health benefits. They speed up the movement of foods through the colon. They can hold water to generate larger softer stools that can quickly and easily removed, thereby preventing and alleviating constipation and other intestinal disorders, They function like a sponge absorbing water, sweeping stools, bile acids, and other toxic fluids through the bowels. They have been linked to the prevention of colon cancer as well as other types of cancer including lung, breast, and cervical cancer. Scientists suggest that fibers prevent cancer by binding to those carcinogen products commonly found in foods, speeding up their removal, and thereby reducing their contact with the intestinal lining. In addition, foods that are high in fiber: usually low in fat and rich in nutrients such as vitamins C, A, and E, which may be a contributing factor in reducing the risk of that dreadful health condition.

Insoluble fibers may help control weight by adding bulk that fills the stomach and helps control appetite. Since they are also low in fat may be an added benefit that causes weight loss. The best sources of fiber are plant foods rather than supplements which tend to bind with essential nutrients making them less absorbable, and putting you at risk for deficiency. Be sure to drink sufficient water to avoid the risk of intestinal blockage associated with fiber pills. The foods that I enjoy the most for their fibers are bananas, apples, pears, oranges, grapefruits, strawberries, watermelon, apricots, peaches, carrots, tomatoes, lettuce, cucumbers, celery, cabbage, and flaxseeds.

Fiber is not a nutrient, since it passes through the digestive system without breaking down. However, there is no doubt that a diet high in fiber is far superior to the typical American diet loaded with unnatural foods that promote diseases. Experts stipulate that fiber deficiency is the prime cause of many modern-day afflictions, and can cure or prevent most of these health conditions including obesity, intestinal disorders, cancer, diabetes, high blood pressure, and heart and vascular diseases. Consuming more living foods will supply enough fibers to maintain the colon and the body as a whole in a healthy condition.

# WATER

Water is an essential element of life. All living things depend on it for survival. No one can survive on Earth without this precious liquid. Without water, the body is unable to absorb salts or convert sugar into glycogen. Water is present in every cell and body tissue. After all 70 percent of a human body is pure water. You may have witnessed what happen to a plant that is lacking of water. It becomes very dry, wilts, and subsequently dies. The same degenerative process can happen to a human body if deprived of water.

The body requires a steady supply of water to perform a multitude of physiological functions. Water loads the nutrients from the food we eat to the blood, and carries them to each cell. In the process, it removes toxins and waste products from the cells to the lungs, skin, and kidneys to be excreted. It helps solid wastes move throughout the intestines. In addition, it regulates the body temperature and lubricates the joints. Every biological process inside the body requires water, which is why it is extremely vital to consume enough to maintain proper metabolic balance.

However, drinking water will not be sufficient to carry out these various bodily functions efficiently. Plain water does not carry nourishing enzymes and other health-giving nutrients. The body requires pure natural water-filled foods found exclusively in fresh fruits and vegetables for nourishment and cleansing as well. Their distilled-rich nutrient water content fulfills the nutritional requirements of the human system. They contain all the enzymes, vitamins, minerals, carbohydrates, fibers, amino acids, and fatty acids the body needs to maintain wellness. These essential nutrients are carried by the water in fruits and vegetables into the colon where they are absorbed into the bloodstream. The water content of fruits and vegetables also performs the requisite task of cleansing or detoxifying the body. Just as it is necessary to wash the outside of the body, the inner body needs to be washed as well. The body craves water because of its constant need to replace the stagnant and dirty water in the system with clean fresh water to ensure an efficient elimination process.

It is imperative to wash our clothes, car, and home, yet we neglect the crucial need to wash the intestines. We eat in such ways that hamper the body's natural cleansing process. If someone close to you decides not to shower or change clothes for three months, the accumulation of dirt, sweat, dead cells, and the ill-smelling odor that would emanate from that individual will certainly be very offensive. The same process occurs when the colon is not washed regularly. When undigested food residues, body wastes, and dead cell proteins are not washed out of the digestive system, they corrupt and pollute the bloodstream. Years of poor eating habits and failure to wash the toxins out of the colon a contributing factors to obesity, heart disease, cancer, and many other health-threatening conditions.

A dietary regimen that consists mainly of concentrated foods such as animal products, refined starches, and sugars will not only clog the intestines but also the arteries. There is no other potent fluid than the distilled nutritional water content of fruits and vegetables that can adequately assist the body in its cleansing function. No vitamin supplements or other man-made laboratory concoctions can duplicate the human body's requirement of rich nutrients and high water content of fresh fruits and vegetables, which is indispensable to achieving weight loss and wellness.

You may probably wonder about the traditional recommendation of drinking eight glasses of water daily. People who eat mainly solid or concentrated foods will feel the need to drink a lot of water simply because they are not getting any from these kinds of foods. However, a diet consisting primarily of raw live foods will supply a substantial amount of water, thereby decreasing the desire to consume much water. However, certain strenuous physical activities, or exposure to sun, heat, or wind, may cause water loss, thereby requiring an increase in water intake.

If you wish to drink water, you should be aware that a pure water supply is unlikely to be available through municipal water, which may contain some potentially hazardous levels of lead and bacteria. Even chlorine and fluoride are considered to be a serious threat to health. Chlorine, which has been added to the water supply for protection against potentially deadly bacteria, has been proven to produce cancer-causing compounds in the water supply. Fluoride added to water to prevent tooth decay has some negative effects on the teeth and even the bones. Studies suggest that fluoride causes tooth staining, and a decrease in bone mass and strength leading to an increased rate of bone fracture in elderly people. In addition, laboratory tests confirmed that fluoride causes cancer in animals.

The safest alternative is to buy distilled bottled water or a home distilled water device. This process not only purifies water by boiling and condensing it but also removes the heavy metals and inorganic compounds.

Given the need to consume an adequate supply of this vital nutrient to avoid dehydration, you cannot rely on thirst only to determine a water deficit. A lack of perspiration during intense activity and a state of lethargy are warning signs of dehydration. Skimpy urination or smelly dark yellow urine are also strong indications that dehydration is present.

A daily consumption of high-water-content foods will constantly wash the walls of the colon of impacted impurities, regenerate, condition the digestive system, and prevent the accumulation of toxins. Drinking a glass of water with lemon juice upon arising is an excellent tonic. To satisfy the body's requirement for this vital nutrient, it is necessary to eat as many raw foods as possible, consume plenty of fresh fruits and vegetables or juices, and drink water as desired. Ultimately, you will enjoy a vibrant, lively, and refreshed body.

## VITAMINS

Vitamins are organic substances found in various foods. They are required for nearly every bodily function. For instance, they help digest food, fight off infections, and generate new cells. They are important for the health of every organ in humans including the brain, heart, immune, and nervous system. They are very sensitive to heat. Exposure to heat over one hundred twenty degrees destroys them. They are divided into two categories: fat-soluble and water- soluble vitamins.

There are fifteen recognized vitamins of which four, vitamins A, D, E, and, K are fat-soluble. They are stored in the liver and require fat and minerals to be absorbed in the digestive system. A generous supply of these vitamins is found in carrots, squash, sweet potatoes, dark greens like kale, broccoli, nuts, and seeds.

Water-soluble vitamins C and B-complex cannot be stored in the body and thus must be replenished daily. Any excess amount is lost through the urine. They are found in all citrus fruits and fresh green leafy vegetables.

Supplements of fat-soluble vitamins can be toxic and lead to various illnesses. A balanced diet consisting of fresh fruits, vegetables, nuts, and seeds will provide a sufficient amount of vitamins in balance amount, thereby eliminating the need for supplement intake.

# MINERALS

Minerals are natural elements originating from the soil in which our food plants are grown. As the plants grow, they absorb and store these elements in their roots, stalks, leaves, and fruits. Minerals are required in sufficient amounts to ensure optimum health. They participate in numerous metabolic reactions that occur throughout the body. Minerals not only make up part of the structural component of body tissues, bones, teeth, and blood cells but are also necessary for proper fluid balance and normal cell and muscle functions.

Essential minerals that are required in the diet include calcium, phosphorus, magnesium, sulfur, sodium, and potassium. Other minerals needed in smaller amounts are called trace minerals including iron, zinc, iodine, copper, manganese, selenium, and chromium. Sources of minerals are fruits, leafy green vegetables, nuts, and seeds.

Vitamins and minerals play a major role in maintaining good health. They are essential for proper cell metabolism. Incorporating an adequate amount of vitamins and minerals can promote psychological well-being, longevity, and chronic disease prevention.

# FAT

**F**at and cholesterol are usually the main concerns of many health-conscious consumers since it has become common knowledge that diets high in fat and cholesterol can be damaging to health. There are so many confusing terms and controversial reports on that subject that people are often baffled about how to manage their dietary diet fat consumption. The fact is the amount and the type of fat in your does have a serious impact on your state of health. Fats consumption has been linked to obesity, clogged arteries, heart disease, cancer, and numerous degenerative conditions like diabetes, high blood pressure, arthritis, and many others. In a desperate effort to prevent those dreadful conditions, medical experts and the food industry have been advocating fat-free products and a low-fat diet. Consumers should be encouraged to increase their intake of essential fatty acids and be advised of the best source of fats and their role in maintaining health.

Fats are essential for normal bodily functions. They are an important building block for all cell membranes and hormone production. They are stored for body insulation and as a major source of energy. They are also needed to replenish the fatty outer layer around the nerves, pad joints, and

84

organs, and assist in the absorption of fat-soluble vitamins (A, D, E, K). The body requires a small percentage of fat in the diet to supply essential fatty acids which are vital to the health and proper function of every living cell. They cannot be produced by the body and must be derived exclusively from plant foods. Fat can be saturated or unsaturated.

Saturated fats are primarily found in all animal foods and dairy products. Plant sources include avocado, cocoa, and coconut. They remain solid at room temperature and tend to stimulate the body's production of cholesterol increasing the blood cholesterol level. Fats from animal sources are unnecessary for human survival. They have such a damaging effect on the heart and arteries and should be restricted from your diet. There are numerous of medical evidence to support the link between a high fat intake from animal sources and the epidemic of degenerative diseases.

Unsaturated fats are found in many plant foods. They are generally liquid at room temperature. They are the body's main source of essential fatty acids, which are necessary for the proper function of the immune and nervous system, and the glow of skin, nails, and hair. The body cannot produce the essential fatty acids that must come from our diet. Their availability depends on the fats not being processed, heated, partially or fully hydrogenated. Unfortunately, mass commercial refinement of these fats destroys the essential fatty acids, causing a rather severe deficiency, contributing to allergies, acne, rashes, brittle nails, dry skin and hair. Refined oils are unnatural, devitalized, and toxic to the human system. After all, human is the only specie that squeezes com, olives, or sunflower seeds to extract their oil. Medical studies indicate that heated fats are carcinogenic, thus, their consumption may promote the growth of certain forms of cancers. Consequently, their antioxidant properties are destroyed making them prone to rancidity and damaging health.

Vegetable oils undergo a process known as hydrogenation that makes them more solid at room temperature and resistant to rancidity. This procedure causes the unsaturated fatty acids not only to become saturated but also to alter their chemical structure. These altered fats generate substances known as trans-fatty acids that act like saturated fats in the body which does not have the digestive capacity to utilize them. Consequently, they poison the body posing serious health risks.

The most alarming nutritional problem in our society is the overconsumption of processed fats and refined oils. Consumers are not even aware of the amount of processed fats consumed daily. Hydrogenated fats are used in every processed food including margarine, candies, cookies, cakes, crackers, chips, breads, peanut butter, mayonnaise, salad dressing, and so many other foods. It is estimated that Americans consume 35 to 40 percent of their daily calories in the form of saturated fats. Statistics have shown that populations that consume a diet high in saturated fats have the highest rate of heart disease. Conversely, a low- fat diet is associated with a lower incidence of heart disease.

It is important to be aware that all oils are 100 percent pure fat. The bottom line is quite simple. Oil should be used sparingly. Nevertheless, health-conscious consumers will always consume unheated natural fats from plant sources rather than processed or animal sources. The body's needs for essential fatty acids, linoleic and linolenic acids, can be met by eating avocado, nuts, and seeds in their raw natural state. Although these foods have some saturated fats, plant foods not only have the highest quality of essential fatty acids but also contain no cholesterol, which makes them the ideal source.

Dietary essential fatty acids are converted to hormone-like substances known as prostaglandins that regulate a host of bodily functions. These nutrients have been extensively studied for their beneficial effects on various health conditions. They help lower cholesterol and high blood pressure to prevent heart and vascular diseases. They can alleviate many inflammatory conditions including arthritis, psoriasis, and eczema. They help the kidneys remove sodium and water since water retention causes swollen ankles, overweight, and pre-menstrual symptoms. They can relieve asthma and allergy symptoms, improve visual function, and increase vitality. They are a useful supplement for the control of diabetes.

Our modern-day deficiency of essential fatty acids and the resulting health afflictions can be relieved by organic unrefined flaxseed oil, which is considered to be very beneficial to numerous health dilemmas. It contains some unique properties that have been proven to have many positive effects on the body. Researchers have isolated substances known as phytoestrogens, which are potent antioxidants that can inhibit cancer. These compounds act as a weak form of estrogen that has been proven to reduce hot flashes symptoms during menopause. Many women who are concerned about the negative side effects of the standard hormone replacement therapy are turning to flax and soy as well for a more natural food-based therapy. Flax is also famous for its ability to make the skin velvety soft, and the nails and hair stronger and healthier.

When considering a dietary essential fatty acids source, flaxseed is a very healthy choice. It is recognized as nature's richest source of omega-3 and omega-6 fatty acids. These natural plant substances have created a great deal of interest in the treatment and prevention of many health problems. Scientific research supports its use in promoting optimal health. Whole flaxseed, with its mild nutty flavor, deserves a place alongside your kitchen staples. It is sold in most health food stores. Pre-ground seeds should not be used, because as soon as they are chattered, the highly unsaturated oil inside oxidizes and spoils quickly. The easiest way to use them is to add them to your fruit smoothies. To reap the full benefits of flax's vital functions, other essential nutrients such as proteins, vitamins, and minerals must be present in sufficient amounts.

# CHOLESTEROL

C holesterol is a soft, waxy, yellowish, substance that is produced by the liver. It is an essential component of the cells. The body needs cholesterol to build cell membranes, sex hormones, bile acids, and vitamin D. It is present in every part of the body including the muscles, skin, liver, intestines, heart, brain, and nervous system, etc. The blood cholesterol level is affected not only by the saturated fat and cholesterol in the diet but also by the cholesterol the body produces. The hard truth is eating foods rich in cholesterol, such as animal products, eggs, and dairy products increases the liver's production of cholesterol. Humans do not need to consume any dietary cholesterol, since the body produces the exact amount needed to perform the various cholesterol- related tasks. The cholesterol in the food you ingest is pure excess that is promptly absorbed from the intestinal tract, which causes a serious health threat since the body can only dispose of a small amount. What happens when there is a surplus in the body?

The amount of what the body needs is then deposited in some body tissues such as the skin, abdominal organs, and the lining of the arteries forming plaques constricting the blood circulation. The extent of the accumulation is reflected in the cholesterol level of the blood. A high level of blood cholesterol leads to atherosclerosis or narrowing of the arteries causing less blood to flow to the heart, thereby increasing the risks of developing heart diseases.

To prevent or even eradicate the tremendous ill effects associated with cholesterol, it would be wise to completely remove all animal products from the diet. Fortunately, most foods that are saturated fats are also high in cholesterol. Thus, by avoiding foods high in saturated fats, you I will be able to get rid of cholesterol in your diet. The exclusion of foods high in cholesterol is rather a simple task. Just think of animals. Cholesterol is exclusively derived from all animal products including beef, poultry, pork, fish, eggs, milk, butter, cheese, ice cream, and yogurt. However, if you choose to consume these foods, the most effective defense against high blood cholesterol levels is to adopt a dietary lifestyle that is very low in saturated fats and cholesterol. That means eating fewer animal products and more live foods. After all, your daily food choices will determine whether the body you live in is lean, energetic, and healthy.

# PROTEIN

P rotein is the most fascinating topic in science and nutrition. Everyone seems to be overly concerned about getting enough of it. When people find out that I do not eat animal products and cooked foods, the most frequent questions raised are: Where do you get your proteins? What do you eat? Don't you find it difficult to eat out? I was amazed to find out how obsessive people can be about protein. That obsession even translates to the fear of not getting enough when in reality they are consuming too much. It also indicates their lack of concern about the ill effects of the digestion of meat proteins on health, and the regeneration of cells and body tissues. I have also noticed that while people are conditioned to eat concentrated proteins, yet, they remain rather confused and misinformed about that nutrient. The fact that there are so many conflicting data further complicates its understanding. Consequently, society tends to make the wrong dietary choices as to the amount and the kind of protein needed to maintain health.

Protein is essential in our diet. It is the building block materials that make and repair muscles, bones, blood vessels, hormones, skin, hair, and nails. It is the main component of the cell nucleus and along with fat is incorporated into the membrane part of every cell. The basic structure of a protein is a chain of twenty-two amino acids, which are compounds containing carbon, hydrogen, oxygen, and nitrogen. The body can produce fourteen of these amino acids. But the eight essential ones must be obtained from foods. All plant foods have substantial amounts of the essential amino acids. Herbivore animals, such as cows, eat plants and store the amino acids in their muscles, thus raw meats are concentrated in proteins.

The human body cannot handle a complete meat protein. The digestive system must break it down into its components of amino acids, which the body uses to build the protein it needs. This is a rather complex process of disintegration requiring the digestive system to overwork strenuously. The digestion of animal foods requires more time and energy than any other food. They take two to three days to go through the intestinal tract because they lack the fiber necessary for efficient digestion. You can visualize what happens to a piece of muscle stored in a dark, moist, and hot place for a few days; it quickly decomposes. When that decayed food is finally excreted, you can smell that offensive putrid odor. Corrupted foods in the digestive system are toxic and acidic contributing to intestinal disorders. Their absorption stresses the body leading to obesity, chronic fatigue, and premature aging. In addition, extensive data indicate the link between concentrated meat proteins and various degenerative conditions such as heart and vascular diseases, diabetes, kidney failure, cancer, osteoporosis, arthritis, other common ailments. cancer, and many

Animal flesh infuses the bloodstream with a toxic dose of excess proteins and fats that impair the various physiological functions of the body. When excess carbohydrates or fats are consumed, the body can store the extra energy as fat. Yet, the human system is unable to store extra protein, thereby causing the digestive system to overwork to break it down into various components. This process generates urea, creatinine, and uric acid that must be eliminated through the kidneys. These toxic substances create an acid condition in the blood, which leaches calcium from the bones. The calcium is then excreted in the urine along with the protein by-products.

Part of the meat and milk protein myth is that they are necessary to build or maintain strong healthy bones and teeth. However, it is the overconsumption of animal-concentrated proteins that causes significant loss of calcium causing the so-called osteoporosis, which has reached epidemic proportions in this country. The milk industry has managed to perpetuate the belief that milk protein is not only the perfect food for humans from birth to old age, but also without it we are condemned to develop calcium deficiency. A look at nature reveals that herbivores such as horses, cows, or elephants get their calcium from plants to build and maintain their enormous bone structure. Humans can also get theirs from plants. Dairy products are loaded with saturated fats, casein, pesticides, and traces of antibiotics, penicillin, and phosphate that make them toxic and, thus unfit for human consumption. Milk, the most mucus-forming food, was solely intended by nature to nurture a baby calve into developing huge bones. The great percentage of casein content in cow's milk, which is used to manufacture the toughest clue, makes it difficult to digest and assimilate by the human body. It clogs the system with toxic mucus that is stored in the sinus cavities, throat, lungs and other vital organs of the body leading to various allergic and inflammatory reactions including chronic runny nose, allergies, asthma, bronchitis, and many other common health conditions. In addition, surveys indicate that the nations with the highest rate of dairy consumption have also the highest incidences of osteoporosis.

The best sources of calcium include fresh leafy vegetables, raw nuts and seeds, and concentrated fruits such as apricots, figs, dates, and prunes. Plant proteins are less concentrated and since they are mixed with oils and complex carbohydrates, they are easier to absorb into the intestines.

When the nutritional aspects of animal proteins are carefully analyzed, their consumption is not worth all the health risks associated with them. The primary purpose of eating any foods relates to their basic nutritional value. Animal proteins do not provide any benefit whatsoever, they can only disintegrate human health. Energy is the essence of life. Proteins do not provide fuel or energy to the body; it is used for enzyme production and the maintenance of other proteins in the body. Carbohydrates and fats supply fuel to the body for energy. A protein meal loaded with fats and excess proteins takes away so much energy from the body leading to the lethargic state that meat eaters are so accustomed to. Whereas a life food meal leaves you feeling refreshed, alive, and energetic for hours. The body's negative health reactions to flesh foods indicate that humans are not suitable for its consumption.

Human physiology is not designed for animal flesh consumption. Carnivores are ideally equipped to acquire and digest meat. They are armed with a strong wide jaw, and long sharp pointed fangs that are used to hunt, kill their prey, and tear their flesh into chunks to swallow. A man who ventures into the wilderness with no weapons in search of food will be more likely to fall victim to his prey.

Mankind is rather suited for food gathering; we have deft fingers for plucking fruits from trees, and short flat grinding molar teeth to eat plant foods that need to be masticated and mixed with the digestive enzymes in his saliva. Meat eater's saliva is acid and adapted to digest animal protein. Our saliva is alkaline and contains ptyalin to predigest plant foods.

There are other striking differences in the digestive system. The stomach of carnivores contains 20 times more hydrochloric acid necessary to digest excess proteins. Their intestinal tract, which is 3 times the length of the body, is structured for decayed meat to pass quickly out of the colon. The human intestinal tract, which measures about 12 times the length of the body's trunk, is designed to hold plant foods high in fiber that can go through the intestines slowly until the nutrients are absorbed. The liver of a carnivore can eliminate a substantial amount of uric acid. Meat protein releases a great amount of uric acid in the system, which is harmful and poisonous to humans who lack the enzyme uricase necessary to neutralize or break it down. The liver of a human can only expel a small amount of uric acid. Thus, the excess is stored and accumulated in the muscles forming small uric acid crystals that cause extensive damage to the nerves leading to conditions such as rheumatism or neuritis.

If mankind were physiologically adapted to ingest meat, he would be effectively equipped to devour and digest it just like real carnivores. The structure of the digestive system was intended to digest plant foods, which are high in fiber, and complex carbohydrates, and contain a modest amount of protein. In addition, we are not even psychologically adapted to consume meat. I wonder how many of us get excited and hungry when we see a cow or a chicken. Unlike carnivores, humans does not have the innate desire for fresh, raw, bloody flesh. For most people, the thought of putting raw muscles in their mouths is very sickening and repugnant. Not to mention the insane idea of going to the wilderness with no tools or weapons and trying to capture a cow for dinner. Can you envision a man jumping on a wild caw, striking it to death, tearing it apart with his teeth, swallowing the warm guts, and flesh voraciously, and licking the blood delightfully? Well, this is a very repulsive scenery. Yet, the idea of eating an apple, a banana, or a raw vegetable salad is strongly appealing and natural to humans. Since we did not evolve as carnivores, one must wonder why we eat flesh foods. Why as a modern society do, we continue to indulge in foods that have enormous devastating effects on our bodies? Why so many people are addicted to animal proteins?

Custom and conditioning are the two reasonable justifications. Flesh consumption is a custom that has been passed on from generation to generation for years a practice that has rarely been questioned by society. Mankind's taste and preference for animal flesh has become a custom. He likes and takes pleasure from eating it without attempting to find out whether or not its consumption is beneficial or damaging to health, and ultimately suffers the consequences associated with meat indulgence. Our taste for flesh foods floods our system with protein and fat that not only make us sick but also set up the stage for degenerative

Society has also been conditioned to believe that animal foods are the most ideal source of protein. This belief is partly due to the research that supports most of the dietary information available to the public. They are funded by powerful organizations that are determined to maximize profits at the expense of the public's health. Through advertising, they successfully managed to preserve the belief that eating a great deal of protein will build a strong body. This is ludicrous, when in fact eating meat does the opposite. A quick look at the animal kingdom reveals that the strongest and biggest animals such as elephants, horses, bulls, or cows eat grasses and leaves. Even those animals that are physiologically similar to humans such as the gorilla, which is famous for its unbelievable strength eat fruits and vegetation. These herbivores get all their proteins and strength by eating plants, which contain substantial amounts of amino acids.

There are no essential nutrients in animal foods required for human strength that cannot be acquired from plant foods. There is no logical explanation as to why we cannot get our supply of amino acids by consuming live foods. The anatomy of the human digestive system is ingeniously designed to digest plant foods, which contain all the essential nutrients required to maintain good health. The consumption of a variety of fruits and vegetables sufficiently meet the protein need of most people. However, when extra protein is required for muscle building, it is necessary to consume raw nuts and seeds. They have many added benefits; they are very low in saturated fats and contain no cholesterol. They also provide fiber and essential fatty acids, which are not available in meat proteins.

Part of the protein myth is the idea of plant protein being incomplete and inadequate. Thus, vegetarians must combine different kinds of foods to get the eight essential amino acids. The basic concept was while meat contains all of the amino acids, plant foods lack one or more amino acids.

This concept has been proven to be misleading. Scientific studies have clearly shown a plant-based diet contains sufficient amounts of amino acids to meet the daily requirements of the human body. Many fruits and vegetables have most of the eight amino acids, yet many foods contain all the eight essential amino acids such as bananas, carrots, cabbage, cauliflower, com, cucumbers, kale, peas, sweet potatoes, tomatoes, nuts, and seeds. The amino acids in live foods are far superior to those from animal sources. They are valuable to humans only when they are unaltered. The cooking process destroys or alters the amino acid chains causing them to become denatured. Consequently, denatured foods are not useful to the body, which processes them as toxins to be eliminated.

The American Dietetic Association stipulated that amino acids from food can combine with amino acids stored in the body. The human body has the most sophisticated structure to ensure that such a vital nutrient like protein is produced continuously with high efficiency. The body has a constant flow of amino acids circulation in the blood. "The body can make up any amino acids missing in a particular meal from its pool of reserves, as long as a variety of foods are included in the diet". Thus, it is unnecessary to burden our dietary lifestyle by combining foods to generate a complete protein meal. Although when planning a nutritious meal, it is a clever dietary strategy to combine a variety of foods to obtain the essential vitamins and minerals, not for the sole purpose of combining proteins.

Let's take a look at another source of protein that is the centerpiece of the breakfast dish of the nation. Perhaps, because eggs are considered a concentrated form of proteins. However, eggs are a health-threatening food that should be eliminated from one's diet. The egg yoke has a high concentration of animal fat that raises cholesterol causing the clogging of the arteries. The highly concentrated protein of the egg white increases the risk of calcium loss. Some egg products are contaminated with salmonella bacteria. Infection from these bacteria can cause diarrhea, severe dehydration, infection of the lungs and nervous system, arthritis, and even death. In addition, eggs are full of sulfur, which can cause tremendous strain and damage to the liver and kidneys as well.

Bear in mind that during the cooking process, the heat destroys most of the amino acids. Thus, what you have left on your plate is a curdle substance that is more noxious rather than nutritious. Eggs are primarily designed for the reproduction of baby chickens, not for human breakfast. The truth is, that the egg is a repugnant substance that corrupts sand toxifies the digestive system. The marvelous human body needs to be nurtured with clean, pure, nutritious live foods and does not require any ill-smelling foods for survival.

Another issue surrounding the meat protein propaganda is vitamin B12. Society has been coerced to believe that the human body requires a great deal of animal proteins to obtain an adequate supply of B12. This psychological myth has been used for years to promote a meat- based diet to maximize the meat industry's profits. After I became a vegan, I was very concerned about my children's risk of developing a B12 deficiency. Eventually, as I gained more knowledge about health and nutrition, I was able to dismiss that myth.

Many of you are probably wondering where animals get their B12 supply. This vitamin is made by bacteria that are common soil organisms. Therefore, B12 is found in small amounts on the surface of fresh garden vegetables. Herbivores such as cows, which are consumed by humans to secure a dose of B12, get theirs by eating plants. Humans can also get this nutrient from the same plant source.

However, B12 is primarily produced in the body by bacteria present in the mouth and intestines. The stomach produces intrinsic factor, which is a substance, that carries the B 12 made by the bacteria in the flora into the colon for absorption. This vitamin is necessary for the formation of red blood cells, healthy nerve function, and the proper use of folic acid. B12 deficiency can cause harmful anemia, a blood disease that leads to nerve tissue degeneration. Symptoms of this condition include chronic fatigue, tingling of the feet or hands, muscle weakness in the legs or arms, memory loss, personality changes, and disorientation. B12 deficiency is rare, but it can occur in people who are not eating the foods containing this particular nutrient. Although the main reason for the deficit is the inability of some people to absorb B12 from their intestines. Old age or other health conditions of the stomach or intestines can hamper the lack of intrinsic factors necessary for absorption.

The theoretical concept that a plant-based diet is deficient in B12 is rather unfounded. The actual requirement of this nutrient is so microscopic that it is measured in micrograms. The Daily Requirement Allowance (RDA) is 2 micrograms. Healthy people store a great amount of B12 in their body tissues and usually carry a five-year supply. On the other hand, flesh-eating individuals are more susceptible to experiencing a B12 deficit, since corruption in the digestive tract may prevent or delay the production of this nutrient. Since B12 deficiency, although unlikely can be serious, some precautionary steps can be taken by consuming more fresh raw garden vegetables or their juices daily.

Many people share the common idea that once they decide to give up red meat; they can indulge in seafood and poultry as a healthier alternative source of protein. They are inclined to believe that red meat is the leading cause of heart disease since it contains more saturated fats than other animal proteins. This concept is erroneous; virtually all animal fleshes contain substantial amounts of saturated fat and cholesterol. It does not make a difference whether that flesh comes from a creature that swims flies, walks on two legs, or wiggles a tail. All animal foods contain excess fats and proteins, therefore, they have the same devastating reactions on the human body. Studies reveal that when beef and pork are substituted for fish or chicken, the blood cholesterol level remains the same.

A lifetime diet centering on animal foods will indeed result in the making of a very sick human being. Be aware that the standard American diet does not promote health. It has rather contributed to an epidemic of degenerative ailments. A staggering number of Americans start experiencing the ill effects of the standard of the American diet by the time they reach their thirties. The ultimate consequences of meat indulgence are degenerative conditions and premature death. Studies reveal that countries that consume copious amounts of animal proteins have the highest rates of death from heart disease, stroke, diabetes, and cancer. Despite all the pieces of evidence that meat proteins are life-threatening, society does not have the wisdom to make a conscious and healthy dietary choice because of the fear of breaking customs and habits. However, these social barriers can indeed be broken since they were not determined by nature. Mankind was distinctively designed to eat live natural foods containing the nutrients needed to sustain a high energy level and ensure the cell regeneration process.

Furthermore, live foods are very low in calories, which are in the form of clean-burning carbohydrates. People who are constantly fighting the battle of the bulge are usually amazed and relieved to find out that when they change to a plant-based diet, they can eat copiously and yet, be able to become slim and energetic. The greatest benefit of live foods is their richness in amino acids, enzymes, vitamins, minerals, fiber, and carbohydrates which are ideal and easier for the body's cells to burn as a source of energy. Eating is one of the most pleasurable sensations in life if only one can indulge in nutritious and delicious foods with no guilt feeling, yet experience the loss of excess body fat and an increase in energy and vitality. Live foods provide that delightful sensation simply because they are the nourishment that nature specifically designed and intended for us to nurture our magnificent bodies. They are easier to digest and contain live, vital, and organic elements that can be readily assimilated by the body. Embracing a raw food dietary lifestyle is living in harmony with nature, which means healthy living.

# DIET AND VIOLENCE

Violence is a terrifying dilemma that has a heavy burden on society since no one can predict or prevent an emotional outburst from occurring. Violence has often been attributed to mental disorders. Subsequently, there are numerous data to support the mind and body connection, but not much attention has been given to the body and mind connection. The physical state of health as a potential cause of violent behavior has rarely been addressed. The correlation between diet and violence has captured my attention as a result of the shouting rampages that have disrupted many schools around the country. Many experts have linked those horrendous behaviors to the violent content of movies and video games. Diet as a contributing factor has never been considered, although, some nutritional studies suggest that food allergy, nutritional deficiencies, and excessive sugar intake are the major sources of mood swings and mental disturbances. These factors can produce a continuous state of inner tension, which affects the nervous system.

A chemical imbalance condition may significantly impair the general thought and emotional reactions of a person. Diet and nutritional factors can determine whether an individual is predisposed to mental disturbances. Researchers have found that any nutrient deficiencies can cause mental disturbances. For instance, deficiencies in vitamin C and B complex have been linked to depression and other emotional disorders. They have also discovered that violent people often have elevated copper-zinc and extremely love levels of sodium, potassium, and manganese. Patients with severe antisocial behavior were tested low in copper, zinc, sodium, potassium, and manganese but high in calcium and magnesium. Various mental and emotional disorders have been associated with dietary lifestyles. For instance, manic depression and certain psychotic disorders have been successfully treated with dietary changes.

The nutritional aspects of psychological disorders need to be addressed, since dealing simply with the symptoms will not produce adequate results. Thus, it is crucial to focus on the actual source as well. Nutrient deficiencies can be attributed to the overconsumption of animal products and cooked foods, which are depleted, of the essential elements and the nourishing enzymes that the human system requires to feel satisfied. The consumption of denatured foods causes constant cellular deprivation. The more cooked or unnatural foods we ingest the hungrier and dissatisfied we are. Since our emotional and physical states are interrelated, any physical dissatisfaction may cause various negative emotional reactions such as anxiety, depression, hatred, anger, and aggressiveness. Anyone experiencing this sort of emotional turmoil is like a time bomb ready to explode at any moment.

A continuous intake of animal proteins, refined sugar, and processed and cooked foods that are poorly digested produces toxic wastes that are absorbed into the bloodstream. Toxicity creates an acid pH level in the system that can contribute to impulsive, unruly, and violent behavior. Whereas a dietary lifestyle of mainly living foods generates an alkaline pH level which contributes to a more assertive, friendly, calm, social, and alert state of mind. Toxic people are more inclined to violence and can be a potential threat to others, while people who enjoy wellness are less likely to harm others.

Toxicity in the body reflects on the mind's ability to function effectively. The brain cells depend on the blood for fresh oxygen; thus, they must be affected by the foods we eat since they determine rather the blood is acid or alkaline. Brain cells that are nourished by toxic or acidic blood may hurt thoughts, emotions, and character as well. Just as alcohol or drug overdoses can incapacitate the mind, toxicity in the blood can have the same adverse impact. It is a fact that nerves spread out from the brain to every part of the body. Therefore, it is certainly beneficial to cleanse or detoxify the body by keeping the colon in a pristine and healthy condition to maintain mental clarity. Removing or cleansing the debris and toxic substances from the system and nourishing it with vital organic atoms of fresh raw foods have been shown to produce beneficial effects in many cases of chronic mental and physical symptoms. A body that is well nourished generates a physical sense of satisfaction and serenity, which is reflected in the emotional state. Only live foods supply the blood with the required nutrients that can help keep the mind clear, positive, alert, and sharp.

I truly believe that parents should bring up their children on a natural diet. They should learn from childhood the various functions of human anatomy and how to take care of their body the way nature intended them to be. Eventually, they will be spared most of the physical and mental diseases. They should know that there is no mystery about the cause of most ailments and that nature has provided all the resources to prevent them. They must also be aware that when the body is nurtured with live foods, they will grow into more healthy, clever, and productive adults, and failure to take proper care of their body will result in sickness, pain, premature aging, and death. I am certain that if children were allowed to grow up with a natural diet of living foods, they would develop a deeper appreciation, love, and closeness to nature. Consequently, they will have more respect and concern for injury to humans and animals as well. They will mature to be kind, loving, and gentle human beings.

Recent surveys indicate that Americans consume less than 18% of fresh live foods. There is a possibility that the quality of food consumption may have a serious impact on the rate of violence in a given society. Animal proteins and cooked foods inflict extensive damage not only to the body but also to the mind as well. They are depleted of the nutrients and the vital enzymes that can meet the human body's nutritional requirements at the cellular level. Their consumption results in toxic, ill, and violent-prone individuals. The accumulation of toxic waste and acidity in the system can severely compromise one's emotional state. The elimination of toxic denatured foods on the diet, and the increased intake of fresh live foods will supply the body the essential nutrients, generate a sense of satisfaction, and promote a positive mental attitude and respect for human lives. A strong and healthy body reflects a strong and healthy mind.

# THE ROLE OF EXERCISE

**P**hysical activities play a significant role in maintaining good health. The hard truth is without exercise the body tends to deteriorate faster despite a healthy dietary lifestyle. Yet, if you are on the (SAD) standard American diet you are not only subjected to a diet deficiency but also an exercise deficiency. Activity is the law of nature. Let's take a look at the animal kingdom. All animal species perform some type of physical activity. They walk, run, jump, climb, swim, fly, or squirm. Human needs to be physically active as well to build muscle strength and stimulate the heart and circulatory systems. Exercise floods your system with fresh oxygen leading to a surge of energy and allowing the body to function efficiently. It is the most effective and powerful aid for weight loss.

Exercising to promote wellness is quite simple. Unlike dieting, there are no restrictions or specific instructions to follow. Depending on your health condition you might want to have a stress test to determine the type of exercise that is safe and appropriate for you. The next step is to select a fitness activity that you feel comfortable with, and then commit yourself to it. Of course, if you have been sedentary for years, you will feel some discomfort and perhaps some pain. It is important to learn to listen to your body. Always choose a workout that you enjoy and will not cause pain or injury to your body

Aerobic exercises such as walking, jogging, cycling, or swimming strengthen your cardiovascular system, improve your muscle tone, and maintain bone density. Walking is the easiest, safest, and fastest way to get fit since it brings most of the body into action. Yet, you do not need your doctor's approval to start a walking program. A daily thirty minutes walk is an excellent start-up that provides fresh air and sunshine which are two vital life forces on Earth. It will also promote an increase of endorphin, a brain chemical that has a positive effect on mood. Twenty minutes of aerobic activity will release enough endorphins to clear the mind and create a feeling of ecstasy that lasts for hours. Another great benefit of exercise is the promotion of healthy perspiration that allows the skin to perform its natural function of eliminating impurities and toxins.

Moderate exercise is a powerful therapeutic aid to manage the so-called diabetic condition. In many cases, it may help eliminate the need for insulin and oral drugs. It helps keep the blood fluid, thereby preventing small clots from blocking the tiny vessels that nourish the eyes and kidneys. This kind of blockage may cause severe damage leading to blindness or kidney failure. In addition, exercise clears the blood glucose. The cells of exercising muscles can extract glucose from the blood more efficiently than inactive muscle cells.

Flexibility, fitness, and physical endurance can be achieved only through exercise. The muscles must be continually used to remain toned, firm, and strong otherwise you lose them. This is the only way to preserve your youthful body shape, experience vitality, or regain your state of health. The flexibility you will acquire from daily stretching will relieve stiffness thereby causing your muscles and joints to become pliable. It may seem to be a formidable task for some people, yet the benefits are so rewarding. The sooner you start, the quicker you will improve your overhaul physical health and well-being, and perhaps recapture the strength, vigor, and self-confidence of youth and be ready to face new challenges.

There are many ways to incorporate a fitness routine into your lifestyle. However, you are the only one who can make the decision, the time, and the commitment to a particular fitness program. Although, once you start enjoying and experiencing the overwhelming benefits associated with exercise, it will undoubtedly become part of your daily routines.

Regular fitness workouts will give you the strength, stamina, and energy to lead a productive life. It is undoubtedly a lifetime habit that provides a long, healthy, and vigorous life. Based on my personal experience, I realize that a perfect state of health can be achieved through daily physical activities combined with the consumption of natural living foods and a positive state of mind.

# CONCLUSION

The world is saturated with nutritional propaganda designed to maximize profits at the expense of the customer's health. This is why it is so important to have some basic knowledge of health and nutrition. However, bear in mind that simplicity is the key to excellent health. The simple natural dietary lifestyle that makes you feel great today is the same that will prevent future degenerative health conditions and cure the ailing as well. Living the hygienic way by abiding by the laws of nature is the only way to achieve wellness. For nature is uncompromising. The raw foodist dietary lifestyle is not a diet program. It is merely living in harmony with nature to preserve the body and keep it fresh, healthy, and vibrant throughout a lifetime. Living the natural way is simple healthy living!

# REFERENCES

Abramowski, O.L.M., M.D. A Doctor's Raw Food Cure. Essence of Health, 1999.

Carper, Jean. The Food Pharmacy. Bantam Books, 1988.

Chapa, Deepak, M.D. Alternative Medicine. Future Medicine Publishing, Inc., 1994.

Diamond, Harvey, and Marilyn. Fit for Life. Warner Books, Inc., 1987.

Graham, Douglas N., D.C. Nutrition and Athletic Performance, 1999.

Heinerman, John. Encyclopedia of Healing Juices. Parker Publishing Company, 1994.

Klaper, Michael, M.D. Vegan Nutrition: Pure and Simple. Gentle World, Inc., 1997.

Krok, Morris. Amazing New Health System. Health Seekers International, 1978.

Krok, Morris. Golden Path to Rejuvenation. Essence of Health, 1974.

McDougal, John A., M.D. The McDougal Program. Penguin Books
USA Inc., 1990.

Robbins, John. Diet for a New World. Avon Books, 1992.

Walker, N.W., D.Sc. Become Younger. Norwalk Press, 1949

Walker, N.W., D.Sc. Fresh Vegetables and Fruit Juices. Norwalk Press. 1936.

Walker, N.W., D.Sc, Colon Health. Norwalk Press, 1979

Whitaker, Julian M., M.D. Reversing Diabetes. Warner Books, INC. 1987